Epidemiology, Virulence Factors and Antimicrobial Resistance in *Staphylococcus aureus*

Epidemiology, Virulence Factors and Antimicrobial Resistance in *Staphylococcus aureus*

Guest Editor

Maria de Lourdes Ribeiro de Souza da Cunha

MDPI

Basel • Beijing • Wuhan • Barcelona • Belgrade • Novi Sad • Cluj • Manchester

Guest Editor
Maria de Lourdes Ribeiro de Souza da Cunha
Department of Genetics, Microbiology and Immunology
São Paulo State University (UNESP)
Botucatu
Brazil

Editorial Office
MDPI AG
Grosspeteranlage 5
4052 Basel, Switzerland

This is a reprint of the Special Issue, published open access by the journal *Antibiotics* (ISSN 2079-6382), freely accessible at: https://www.mdpi.com/journal/antibiotics/special_issues/AR_Staphylococcus_aureus.

For citation purposes, cite each article independently as indicated on the article page online and as indicated below:

Lastname, A.A.; Lastname, B.B. Article Title. *Journal Name* **Year**, *Volume Number*, Page Range.

ISBN 978-3-7258-5155-3 (Hbk)
ISBN 978-3-7258-5156-0 (PDF)
https://doi.org/10.3390/books978-3-7258-5156-0

Contents

About the Editor

Maria de Lourdes Ribeiro de Souza da Cunha

Maria de Lourdes Ribeiro de Souza da Cunha, PhD in Tropical Diseases (1998), Associate Professor at São Paulo State University (UNESP), Botucatu, SP, Brazil (2012), is a biologist with main research interests in Microbiology, focusing on Bacteriology, acting on the following subjects: *Staphylococcus aureus*, Coagulase-Negative *Staphylococci* (CoNS), epidemiology, virulence factors, biofilms, enterotoxins, and antimicrobial resistance. She is currently a Senior Professor at the Department of Genetics, Microbiology and Immunology, Institute of Biosciences, São Paulo State University (UNESP), Botucatu, SP, Brazil. She is a scientific reference in *Staphylococcus*, with 56 research projects supported for the São Paulo Research Foundation (FAPESP) and Scholarship in Research Productivity of the National Council for Scientific and Technological Development (CNPq) since 2009. She is the author of more than 100 papers in international peer-reviewed journals, 4 books, and more than 20 chapters in books.

antibiotics

MDPI

Editorial

Epidemiology, Virulence Factors, and Antimicrobial Resistance in *Staphylococcus aureus*

Maria de Lourdes Ribeiro de Souza da Cunha †

Department of Genetics, Microbiology and Immunology, Institute of Biosciences, São Paulo State University (UNESP), Botucatu 18618-691, SP, Brazil; mlrs.cunha@unesp.br
† Senior Professor UNESP.

Serious infections caused by bacteria that are resistant to commonly used antibiotics have become a global health problem in the 21st century. An important example is the methicillin-resistant *Staphylococcus aureus* (MRSA), which poses a serious threat to public health worldwide because of the rapid spread and diversification of pandemic clones, which are characterized by increasing virulence and antimicrobial resistance [1].

Antibiotic resistance, which was initially a problem faced by hospital settings associated with an increased number of hospital-acquired infections, usually in critically ill and immunocompromised patients, has now spread to the wider community, causing serious illness in previously healthy and conventionally non-vulnerable patients [2]. In the case of community-acquired infections, population characteristics, living conditions, agglomerations, underlying diseases, injectable drug use, the presence of insulin-dependent diabetes, and the frequency of antibiotic use contribute to the selection of resistant bacteria. Furthermore, we continue to fail to contain the spread of resistance genes, compromising community healthcare. Community-associated (CA)-MRSA usually occurs in individuals who have not been hospitalized or undergone medical procedures such as dialysis, surgery, or catheterization in the year prior to infection, all of which are common factors in hospital-acquired MRSA (HA-MRSA) infections [3].

Infections caused by *S. aureus* are usually severe because of the production of various virulence factors, including extracellular enzymes, cytolytic toxins, and superantigen toxins. The arsenal of virulence factors of *S. aureus* is extensive; some of them are part of the cell structure itself and others are extracellular factors that are produced during growth and excreted to the extracellular medium. Both types of virulence factors play important roles in the pathogenesis of infection [4].

The typical cultural behaviors of different populations, such as overcrowded living conditions, compromised healthcare, and poor hygiene, may be more relevant in the pathogenesis of some forms of *S. aureus* infections. Within this context, natives undeniably belong to the risk group for carrying resistant microorganisms and are susceptible to both the acquisition and spread of infections [5].

The study by Abraão et al. (2023) investigated the prevalence and risk factors for nasal and oral carriage of methicillin-sensitive *S. aureus* (MSSA) and MRSA among indigenous communities in northern and southeastern Brazil. The authors evaluated genetic diversity, dissemination, virulence factors, and antimicrobial resistance associated with ethnic, demographic, environmental, and behavioral factors. A total of 400 Indians (from near-urban areas and remote hamlets) were screened for *S. aureus* and CA-MRSA colonization. The study revealed a higher prevalence of *S. aureus* carriage among Shanenawa ethnicity individuals (41.1%). Thus, ethnicity appears to be associated with the prevalence of *S. aureus* in

 https://doi.org/10.3390/antibiotics14080792

these populations. CA-MRSA was found in three isolates (0.7%), all of them SCC*mec* type IV. PFGE analysis identified 21 clusters among the *S. aureus* isolates and MLST analysis showed a predominance of sequence type 5 among these isolates.

Considering a completely different perspective, people living with HIV/AIDS must be cited as a risk group. Studies conducted in different countries demonstrated significant colonization of this population with MRSA, a finding that can be attributed in part to their intense contact with health services [6]. In the study by Obanda et al. (2022) investigating abattoir workers, MRSA carriage was higher in HIV-positive individuals (24/89, 27.0%) than in HIV-negative participants (94/648, 14.5%; $p = 0.003$). The prevalence of MRSA carriage (0.4%) identified in that study was low compared to studies conducted with abattoir workers in Europe (5.6%) [7] and the United States (3.6%) [8]. However, the low rate is consistent with another study investigating MRSA carriage in Kenya (0.8%) [9].

Studies found that individuals carrying a high bacterial load have a six times greater risk of developing staphylococcal infection than non-carriers or individuals with a low bacterial load [10]. This phenomenon seems to be even more common among MRSA carriers [11]. Although the nasopharynx is the most consistent site of colonization by *S. aureus* and has been indicated as the most appropriate site for swab sampling, other sites (extra-nasal) can also be colonized. Recent studies demonstrated that a substantial number of individuals, ranging from 7% to 32%, are exclusive *S. aureus* carriers in the oropharynx, suggesting that the inclusion of a throat swab in addition to a nasal swab may be important for the success of surveillance programs [12].

The study by Silva et al. (2022) investigated the prevalence and factors associated with the nasal, oral, and rectal carriage of *S. aureus* and MRSA in bedridden patients and residents of long-term care facilities for the elderly (LTCFs) in Botucatu, SP, Brazil. The prevalence of *S. aureus* and MRSA was 33.6% ($n = 76$) and 8% ($n = 18$), respectively. At the nine LTCFs studied, the prevalence of *S. aureus* ranged from 16.6% to 85.7% and that of MRSA from 13.3% to 25%. The study showed a high prevalence of *S. aureus* among elderly residents of small (<15 residents) and medium-size (15–49 residents) LTCFs, as well as a higher prevalence of MRSA in the oropharynx.

The contributions to this Special Issue on clinical MRSA isolates include the following studies: Boutet-Dubois et al. (2023) described the phenotypic and genotypic evolution of MRSA strains that became resistant to daptomycin (DAP) in two unrelated patients with bacteremia treated with this antibiotic in two hospitals in the South of France. DAP MICs were determined using the broth microdilution method on the pairs of isogenic (DAP-S/DAP-R) *S. aureus* isolated from bloodstream cultures. Whole-genome sequencing was carried out using the Illumina MiSeq Sequencing system. The two cases revealed DAP-R acquisition by MRSA strains within three weeks in patients treated with DAP. The study highlights the non-systematic cross-resistance between DAP and glycopeptides. The use of DAP as first-line therapy at optimal dosages must be considered when patients are at risk of MRSA infection. Moreover, it is crucial to monitor DAP MIC in persistent MRSA bacteremia. Kmiha et al. (2023) studied the genetic lineages, antibiotic resistance genes, and virulence determinants of *S. aureus* isolates from clinical samples of burn patients in Tunisia. All isolates from the clinical samples of burn patients were confirmed as MRSA, with high rates of resistance to ciprofloxacin and gentamicin conferred by different antibiotic resistance genes. The data revealed the presence of resistance genes and a different virulence profile in MRSA isolates. Tălăpan et al. (2023) evaluated the frequency of isolation of *S. aureus* from different pathological samples in Romania in order to establish the ratio of MRSA to MSSA strains and the antibiotic resistance profile of the isolated microorganisms. Up to 39.11% of *S. aureus* strains were resistant to oxacillin (MRSA), with 49.97% being resistant to erythromycin and 36.06% showing inducible resistance to clindamycin. Resistance rates to ciprofloxacin, rifampicin, gentamicin, and trimethoprim-sulfamethoxazole were 9.98%, 5.38%, 5.95%, and 0.96%, respectively. There was no resistance to vancomycin. Between 2017 and 2022, the percentage of MRSA strains decreased from 41.71% to 33.63% but sharply increased to 42.42% in 2021 (the year of the COVID-19 pandemic, when the percentage of strains isolated from lower respiratory tract infections was higher than that of strains isolated from wounds or blood, as in previous years). Quezada-Aguiluz et al. (2022) aimed to detect and characterize resistance to macrolides, lincosamides, and type B streptogramins among HA-MRSA and CA-MRSA isolates collected between 2007 and 2017 within the *S. aureus* surveillance program of the National Institute of Public Health of Chile (ISP). Most of the HA-MRSA isolates (97%) were resistant to clindamycin, erythromycin, azithromycin, and clarithromycin. Among CA-MRSA isolates, 28% were resistant to erythromycin and azithromycin and 25% to clarithromycin. The *ermA* gene was the predominant gene identified among these isolates.

Staphylococcus pseudintermedius is an opportunistic pathogen frequently isolated from canines [13]. Suepaul et al. (2023) focused on isolates obtained from healthy dogs and their owners who presented at clinics for routine veterinary care and used whole-genome sequencing-based analyses for strain comparisons. A total of 25 humans and 27 dogs were sampled at multiple sites, yielding 47 and 45 isolates, respectively. Whole-genome sequence analysis was performed. The virulence content did not provide insights toward a tendency of colonization of humans but supported that there may be differences in the surface proteins between carrier strains and those causing pyoderma. The study identified 13 cases in which humans were infected with strains from the dog they owned.

The cited studies are relevant since they suggest that *S. aureus* carriers are at higher risk of acquiring infection and are an important source of dissemination of bacteria among individuals. A comprehensive approach involving the special populations described above that combines epidemiological strategies with genetic characterization of staphylococci may provide insights into the genesis and dissemination of MRSA strains.

Funding: This research was funded by the National Council for Scientific and Technological Development (CNPq), grant number 303603/2020-8.

Conflicts of Interest: The author declares no conflicts of interest.

List of Contributions:

1. Boutet-Dubois, A.; Magnan, C.; Lienard, A.; Pouget, C.; Bouchet, F.; Marchandin, H.; Larcher, R.; Lavigne, J.-P.; Pantel, A. In Vivo-Acquired Resistance to Daptomycin during Methicillin-Resistant *Staphylococcus aureus* Bacteremia. *Antibiotics* **2023**, *12*, 1647. https://doi.org/10.3390/antibiotics12121647.
2. Suepaul, S.; Stegger, M.; Boyen, F.; Georges, K.; Butaye, P. The Diversity and Zoonotic Potential of *Staphylococcus pseudintermedius* in Humans and Pet Dogs in Trinidad and Tobago. *Antibiotics* **2023**, *12*, 1266. https://doi.org/10.3390/antibiotics12081266.
3. Kmiha, S.; Jouini, A.; Zerriaa, N.; Hamrouni, S.; Thabet, L.; Maaroufi, A. Methicillin-Resistant *Staphylococcus aureus* Strains Isolated from Burned Patients in a Tunisian Hospital: Molecular Typing, Virulence Genes, and Antimicrobial Resistance. *Antibiotics* **2023**, *12*, 1030. https://doi.org/10.3390/antibiotics12061030.
4. Tălăpan, D.; Sandu, A.-M.; Rafila, A. Antimicrobial Resistance of *Staphylococcus aureus* Isolated between 2017 and 2022 from Infections at a Tertiary Care Hospital in Romania. *Antibiotics* **2023**, *12*, 974. https://doi.org/10.3390/antibiotics12060974.
5. Abraão, L.M.; Fortaleza, C.M.C.B.; Camargo, C.H.; Barbosa, T.A.; Pereira-Franchi, E.P.L.; Riboli, D.F.M.; Hubinger, L.; Bonesso, M.F.; Medeiros de Souza, R.; Ribeiro de Souza da Cunha, M.d.L. *Staphylococcus aureus* and CA-MRSA Carriage among Brazilian Indians Living in Peri-Urban Areas and Remote Communities. *Antibiotics* **2023**, *12*, 862. https://doi.org/10.3390/antibiotics12050862.

6. Obanda, B.A.; Gibbons, C.L.; Fèvre, E.M.; Bebora, L.; Gitao, G.; Ogara, W.; Wang, S.-H.; Gebreyes, W.; Ngetich, R.; Blane, B.; et al. Multi-Drug Resistant *Staphylococcus aureus* Carriage in Abattoir Workers in Busia, Kenya. *Antibiotics* **2022**, *11*, 1726. https://doi.org/10.3390/antibiotics11121726.
7. Silva, L.P.; Fortaleza, C.M.C.B.; Teixeira, N.B.; Silva, L.T.P.; de Angelis, C.D.; Ribeiro de Souza da Cunha, M.d.L. Molecular Epidemiology of *Staphylococcus aureus* and MRSA in Bedridden Patients and Residents of Long-Term Care Facilities. *Antibiotics* **2022**, *11*, 1526. https://doi.org/10.3390/antibiotics11111526.
8. Quezada-Aguiluz, M.; Aguayo-Reyes, A.; Carrasco, C.; Mejías, D.; Saavedra, P.; Mella-Montecinos, S.; Opazo-Capurro, A.; Bello-Toledo, H.; Munita, J.M.; Hormazábal, J.C.; et al. Phenotypic and Genotypic Characterization of Macrolide, Lincosamide and Streptogramin B Resistance among Clinical Methicillin-Resistant *Staphylococcus aureus* Isolates in Chile. *Antibiotics* **2022**, *11*, 1000. https://doi.org/10.3390/antibiotics11081000.

References

1. WHO. *Bacterial Priority Pathogens List, 2024: Bacterial Pathogens of Public Health Importance to Guide Research, Development and Strategies to Prevent and Control Antimicrobial Resistance*; World Health Organization: Geneva, Switzerland, 2024.
2. Bellis, K.L.; Dissanayake, O.M.; Harrison, E.M.; Aggarwal, D. Community methicillin-resistant *Staphylococcus aureus* outbreaks in areas of low prevalence. *Clin. Microbiol. Infect.* **2025**, *31*, 182–189. [CrossRef] [PubMed]
3. Tsouklidis, N.; Kumar, R.; Heindl, S.E.; Soni, R.; Khan, S. Understanding the Fight Against Resistance: Hospital-Acquired Methicillin-Resistant *Staphylococcus aureus* vs. Community-Acquired Methicillin-Resistant *Staphylococcus aureus*. *Cureus* **2020**, *12*, e8867. [CrossRef] [PubMed]
4. Touaitia, R.; Mairi, A.; Ibrahim, N.A.; Basher, N.S.; Idres, T.; Touati, A. *Staphylococcus aureus*: A Review of the Pathogenesis and Virulence Mechanisms. *Antibiotics* **2025**, *14*, 470. [CrossRef] [PubMed]
5. Golding, G.R.; Levett, P.N.; McDonald, R.R.; Irvine, J.; Nsungu, M.; Woods, S.; Horbal, A.; Siemens, C.G.; Khan, M.; Ofner-Agostini, M.; et al. Northern Antibiotic Resistance Partnership (NARP). A comparison of risk factors associated with community-associated methicillin- resistant and -susceptible Staphylococcus aureus infections in remote communities. *Epidemiol. Infect.* **2010**, *138*, 730–737. [CrossRef] [PubMed]
6. Hidron, A.I.; Kempker, R.; Moanna, A.; Rimland, D. Methicillin-resistant *Staphylococcus aureus* in HIV-infected patients. *Infect. Drug. Resist.* **2010**, *3*, 73–86. [CrossRef]
7. Van Cleef, B.A.G.L.; Broens, E.M.; Voss, A.; Huijsdens, X.W.; Zuchner, L.; Van Benthem, B.H.B.; Kluytmans, J.A.J.W.; Mulders, M.N.; Van De Giessen, A.W. High prevalence of nasal MRSA carriage in slaughterhouse workers in contact with live pigs in theNetherlands. *Epidemiol. Infect.* **2010**, *138*, 756–763. [CrossRef] [PubMed]
8. Leibler, J.H.; Jordan, J.A.; Brownstein, K.; Lander, L.; Price, L.B.; Perry, M.J. *Staphylococcus aureus* nasal carriage among beefpacking workers in a MidwesternUnited States slaughterhouse. *PLoS ONE* **2016**, *11*, e0148789. [CrossRef] [PubMed]
9. Aiken, A.M.; Mutuku, I.M.; Sabat, A.J.; Akkerboom, V.; Mwangi, J.; Scott, J.A.G.; Morpeth, S.C.; Friedrich, A.W.; Grundmann, H. Carriage of *Staphylococcus aureus* in Thika Level 5 Hospital, Kenya: A cross-sectional study. *Antimicrob. Resist. Infect. Control.* **2014**, *3*, 22. [CrossRef] [PubMed]
10. Tong, S.Y.; Chen, L.F.; Fowler, V.G., Jr. Colonization, pathogenicity, host susceptibility, and therapeutics for Staphylococcus aureus: What is the clinical relevance? *Semin Immunopathol.* **2012**, *34*, 185–200. [CrossRef] [PubMed]
11. Pimenta Rodrigues, M.V.; Fortaleza, C.M.; Souza, C.S.; Teixeira, N.B.; Cunha, M.L. Genetic Determinants of Methicillin Resistance and Virulence among *Staphylococcus aureus* Isolates Recovered from Clinical and Surveillance Cultures in a Brazilian TeachingHospital. *IRSN. Microbiol.* **2012**, *17*, 975143. [CrossRef]
12. Hamdan-Partida, A.; Sainz-Espuñes, T.; Bustos-Martínez, J. Characterization and persistence of Staphylococcus aureus strains isolated from the anterior nares andthroats of healthy carriers in a Mexican community. *J. Clin. Microbiol.* **2010**, *48*, 1701–1705. [CrossRef] [PubMed]
13. Fàbregas, N.; Pérez, D.; Viñes, J.; Cuscó, A.; Migura-García, L.; Ferrer, L.; Francino, O. Diverse Populations of *Staphylococcus pseudintermedius* Colonize the Skin of Healthy Dogs. *Microbiol. Spectr.* **2023**, *11*, e0339322. [CrossRef] [PubMed]

antibiotics

MDPI

Article

In Vivo-Acquired Resistance to Daptomycin during Methicillin-Resistant *Staphylococcus aureus* Bacteremia

Adeline Boutet-Dubois [1], Chloé Magnan [1], Alexi Lienard [2], Cassandra Pouget [1], Flavien Bouchet [3], Hélène Marchandin [4], Romaric Larcher [5], Jean-Philippe Lavigne [1,*] and Alix Pantel [1]

1 VBIC, INSERM U1047, Department of Microbiology and Hospital Hygiene, University of Montpellier, CHU Nîmes, 30029 Nîmes, France; adeline.dubois@chu-nimes.fr (A.B.-D.); chloe.magnan@chu-nimes.fr (C.M.); cassandra.pouget@chu-nimes.fr (C.P.); alix.pantel@chu-nimes.fr (A.P.)
2 Laboratory of Medical Biology, CH Bassin de Thau, 34207 Sète, France; alienard@ch-bassindethau.fr
3 Department of Internal Medicine-Infectiology, CH Bassin de Thau, 34207 Sète, France; fbouchet@ch-bassindethau.fr
4 HydroSciences Montpellier, Department of Microbiology and Hospital Hygiene, University of Montpellier, CNRS, IRD, CHU Nîmes, 30029 Nîmes, France; helene.marchandin@umontpellier.fr
5 Department of Infectious Diseases, CHU Nîmes, 30029 Nîmes, France; romaric.larcher@chu-nimes.fr
* Correspondence: jean.philippe.lavigne@chu-nimes.fr; Tel.: +33-466683202

Abstract: Daptomycin (DAP) represents an interesting alternative to treat methicillin-resistant *Staphylococcus aureus* (MRSA) infections. Different mechanisms of DAP resistance have been described; however, in vivo-acquired resistance is uncharacterized. This study described the phenotypic and genotypic evolution of MRSA strains that became resistant to DAP in two unrelated patients with bacteremia under DAP treatment, in two hospitals in the South of France. DAP MICs were determined using broth microdilution method on the pairs of isogenic (DAP-S/DAP-R) *S. aureus* isolated from bloodstream cultures. Whole genome sequencing was carried out using Illumina MiSeq Sequencing system. The two cases revealed DAP-R acquisition by MRSA strains within three weeks in patients treated by DAP. The isolates belonged to the widespread ST5 (patient A) and ST8 (patient B) lineages and were of *spa*-type t777 and t622, respectively. SNP analysis comparing each DAP-S/DAP-R pair confirmed that the isolates were isogenic. The causative mutations were identified in MprF (Multiple peptide resistance Factor) protein: L826F (Patient A) and S295L (Patient B), and in Cls protein: R228H (Patient B). These proteins encoded both proteins of the lipid biosynthetic enzymes. The resistance to DAP is particularly poorly described whereas DAP is highly prescribed to treat MRSA. Our study highlights the non-systematic cross-resistance between DAP and glycopeptides and the importance of monitoring DAP MIC in persistent MRSA bacteremia.

Keywords: daptomycin resistance; *mprF* mutations; *cls* mutation; Methicillin-resistant *Staphylococcus aureus*; whole genome sequencing

1. Introduction

Methicillin-resistant *Staphylococcus aureus* (MRSA) infections represent a major health problem, leading to high morbidity and mortality worldwide [1,2]. MRSA strains are resistant to nearly all β-lactams and several other classes of antibiotics such as aminoglycosides, fluoroquinolones, and tetracyclines, restricting the antimicrobial chemotherapy possibilities against those infections. Glycopeptides have long been considered the first-line therapy for severe MRSA infections [1]. However, new antibiotic solutions have emerged to treat infections due to intermediate or resistant vancomycin *S. aureus*. Daptomycin (DAP) represents an interesting alternative treatment of MRSA [1]. This antibiotic is a calcium-dependent lipopeptide that is increasingly used for the treatment of MRSA bloodstream infections due to higher treatment success rate [3] and reduced risk of mortality compared to vancomycin (VAN) [4].

DAP has been isolated from *Streptomyces roseosporus* [5]. This antibiotic has been approved for use and continues to be considered a mainstay of anti-MRSA treatment [6]. It possesses a cyclic peptide core linked to a fatty acyl chain [7]. Associated with calcium, this DAP-Ca^{2+} complex forms tetramers within the outer leaflet and constitute an amphipathic complex that facilitates oligomerization [8]. Finally, the DAP-Ca^{2+} complex forms micelles, which are able to insert into the cell wall of bacteria and bind to phosphatidylglycerol [9]. Thus, these micelles can disrupt the cytoplasmic membrane of Gram-positive bacteria, involving a depolarization, permeabilization, and ion leakage of the bacterium [10–12]. Moreover, the DAP-Ca^{2+} complex masks the negative charge of lipopeptides increasing its affinity for one of the major anionic phospholipids present in the Gram-positive membranes [13]. Multiple DAP mechanisms of action have been published such as membrane permeabilization, inhibition of cell wall synthesis, physical alteration of membrane curvature and fluidity, and disruption of the peptidoglycan synthesis machinery [10,14–17]. Finally, this antibiotic harbors bactericidal and non-bacteriolytic properties. Based on pharmacokinetic studies, DAP exhibits concentration-dependent killing [18].

DAP-resistance is a rare event. Several explanations have been provided. This resistance is mainly associated with the positively-charged membrane of the cell due to alanylation of teichoic acids and the lysinylation of phosphatidylglycerol in cell membrane, repelling the antibiotic. These modifications change the membrane fluidity and reduce the affinity of cationic antimicrobial peptides [19]. In strains not susceptible to DAP, different studies have documented the presence of mutations in various genes encoding enzymes involved in the phospholipid synthesis and metabolism: *mprF* (multiple peptide resistance Factor), *cls* (cardiolipin synthase), and *pgsA* (phospholipid metabolism). Mutations have also been described into two component systems regulating cell membrane stress and permeability, *walk/walR* (also known as *yycF/yycG*) and *vraS/vraR*. Finally, the upregulation of *dltABCD* transcription contributed to enhance the surface positive charge by teichoic acid D-alanination, as observed with *mprF* mutations [20–23]. However, the in vivo-acquired resistance is rarely described [24–26] and some associations between the resistance to VAN and the decreased susceptibility to DAP have been reported [7]. Here, we described the phenotypic and genotypic evolution of MRSA strains that became resistant to DAP in two unrelated patients with bacteremia under DAP treatment only, in two hospitals in the South of France.

2. Results

2.1. Patient A

The patient was an 81-year-old man followed in Nîmes University Hospital (France) for a lung adenocarcinoma discovered in 2012. The patient had developed cerebral metastasis, and after several anti-cancer chemotherapies and interventions, immunotherapy was initiated in February 2020. On April 2021, the patient presented to the Emergency Department at Nîmes University Hospital with local pain next to his central vascular catheter (Port-a-Cath), implanted on three days after. The home nurse also reported a purulent flow for several days. The patient was apyretic, but bloodstream cultures were performed. They incubated in the Bactec FX system (Becton Dickinson, Franklin Lakes, NJ, USA) and were positive 12 h after collection, with Gram-positive cocci observed on Gram staining. The patient was hospitalized in the Pneumology Unit. The Port-a-Cath was removed after two weeks. A probabilistic intravenous antimicrobial therapy combining DAP with piperacillin/tazobactam (TZP) was initiated. The bacterial culture of the device identified a DAP-susceptible (DAP-S) MRSA (MIC of 0.5 mg/L). TZP was stopped three days after and DAP monotherapy was continued at 10 mg/kg/24 h. Despite correct antimicrobial treatment, bloodstream cultures remained positive for *S. aureus*. After two weeks, an antimicrobial susceptibility testing identified DAP-resistant (DAP-R) MRSA isolates (MIC of 2 mg/L). Antimicrobial therapy was switched to intravenous ceftaroline. The patient died two weeks after in palliative care due to complications of his cancer.

2.2. Patient B

The patient was a 69-year-old man diagnosed with Parkinson disease in 2017. He was first hospitalized in Sète General Hospital (France) in October 2020 for surgical treatment of colorectal anastomosis. In June 2021, the patient was re-hospitalized for restoration of intestinal continuity. This stay was complicated with stercoral peritonitis secondary to suture breakage 5 days after surgery. The intraoperative microbiological cultures showed *Escherichia coli, Proteus mirabilis, Enterococcus faecalis,* and *Enterococcus avium.* An antimicrobial therapy associating TZP to fluconazole was initiated. Two weeks after, an abdominal CT scan highlighted a sub-diaphragmatic collection that was radiologically drained. Empiric intravenous antimicrobial therapy with TZP was prescribed. *E. coli, Enterococcus faecalis, P. mirabilis,* and *Staphylococcus capitis* were isolated. Intravenous antimicrobial treatment was switched to meropenem at 6 g/24 h and DAP at 10 mg/kg/24 h for three weeks. At end of July, antimicrobial therapy was stopped. At the beginning of September 2021, the patient was febrile (39 °C) after removal of the PICC-line and subcutaneous catheter. Bloodstream cultures identified a DAP-S MRSA (MIC of 0.5 mg/L). Intravenous antimicrobial therapy with DAP at 10 mg/kg/24 h was initiated for 14 days. Three weeks after, the patient was febrile again with CRP at 176 mg/L. Bloodstream cultures revealed DAP-R MRSA (MIC of 2 mg/L). Antimicrobial therapy was switched to intravenous ceftaroline and clindamycin intravenous association. There was no relapse, and the patient was transferred to a rehabilitation center.

2.3. Description of the Two DAP-R MRSA Isolates

The main characteristics of the pairs of isogenic (DAP-S/DAP-R) *S. aureus* strains are described in Table 1.

The DAP-S (MIC of 0.5 mg/L) MRSA strain isolated from patient A was susceptible to glycopeptides (VAN, TEI and DAL MICs of 1, 0.5 and 0.06 mg/L, respectively) and to advanced generation cephalosporins (CPT and CBP MICs 0.25 and 1 mg/L, respectively). The isolate was resistant to β-lactams (penicillin G and oxacillin) and fluoroquinolones (ofloxacin). After 21 days of exposure to DAP, the strain was resistant to this antibiotic (MIC of 2 mg/L) but no cross-resistance to glycopeptides was observed (VAN, TEI and DAL MICs of 1, 1 and 0.06 mg/L, respectively).

The DAP-S MRSA (MIC of 0.5 mg/L) isolated from patient B was also susceptible to glycopeptides (VAN, TEI and DAL MICs of 1, 0.5 and 0.06 mg/L, respectively) and to CPT and CBP (MIC of 0.38 and 1.5 mg/L, respectively). The isolate was resistant to rifampicin and fluoroquinolones. After 22-days exposure to DAP, a MRSA isolate was detected also resistant to DAP (MIC of 2 mg/L).

2.4. Whole Genome Analysis of the DAP-S/DAP-R Isolates

The wgMLST analysis showed that MRSA isolates belonged to the widespread ST5 (patient A) and ST8 (patient B) lineages and were of *spa*-type t777 and t622, respectively (Table 1). Genome assembly generated median of 2,817,995 bp in size for isolates from patient A and 2,881,993 bp for isolates from patient B, corresponding to median coverage >97% and 0.030% in gap ratio. Whole genome annotation of *S. aureus* genomes from patient A predicted a median of 32.67% of CG content for A_DAP-S and A_DAP-R. The median coding ratios were 99.88% for both isolates including a median of 2530 and of 2529 coding sequences (CDS), and both 61 tRNA and 12 rRNA, respectively. The annotation for isolates from patient B predicted a median of 32.63% of CG content for B_DAP-S and B_DAP-R. The median coding ratios were 99.85% and 99.81%, including a median of 2617 and 2612 CDS, and both 61 tRNA and 10 rRNA for the two isolates, respectively. SNP analysis comparing each pair of DAP-S/DAP-R isolates from each patient confirmed that the isolates were isogenic. For both patients, we observed only one SNP difference between each isolate across the entire genome.

Table 1. Main characteristics of the two pairs of isogenic (DAP-susceptible/DAP-resistant) *S. aureus* isolates.

Strain	Location	Collection Date	Specimen Type	ST	*spa* Type	MICs Values (mg/L):						Resistance Profile	% Sequence Similarities	Mutation in MprF and Cls Proteins *
						DAP	VAN	TEI	DAL	CPT	CBP			
A_DAP-S	Nîmes	26 April 2021	Blood	5	t777	0.5	1	0.5	0.06	0.25	1	PEN, OXA, OFX	99.96	-
A_DAP-R	Nîmes	16 May 2021	Blood	5	t777	2	1	1	0.06	0.38	1	PEN, OXA, OFX		L826F
B_DAP-S	Sète	3 September 2021	Blood	8	t622	0.5	1	0.5	0.06	0.38	1.5	PEN, OXA, OFX, RIF	99.93	-
B_DAP-R	Sète	26 September 2021	Blood	8	t622	2	1	0.5	0.06	0.38	1.5	PEN, OXA, OFX, RIF		S295L/*R228H*

CBP, ceftobiprole; CPT, ceftaroline; DAL, dalbavancin; DAP, daptomycin; TEI, teicoplanin; VAN, vancomycin.; PEN, Penicillin G, OXA, oxacillin, OFX, ofloxacin, RIF, rifampicin; * mutation in Cls protein is in italic.

2.5. Resistome Profiling of the DAP-S/DAP-R Isolates

The four *S. aureus* isolates were predicted in silico to be resistant to penicillin G, methicillin by the presence of *blaZ* and *mecA* genes. The resistance to ofloxacin was provided by point mutations in DNA gyrase subunit A- (*gyrA*) and topoisomerase IV subunit C (*parC*)- encoding genes harbored in all isolates conferring resistance to fluoroquinolones. Isolates from patient B presented classic mutation (D471E) usually predicted in the *rpoB* gene and involved in rifampicin resistance. Finally, the four isolates had *mepA* gene, which encoded efflux pumps and the two isolates from patient B harbored point mutations in *murA* gene, which is responsible for the early rate-limiting step in cell wall synthesis.

2.6. Virulome of the DAP-S/DAP-R Isolates

For the virulome profile of the *S. aureus* isolated from patient A, the whole genome analysis showed that all strains carried enterotoxins- (*sea, sed, sei, sej, sem, sen, seo,* and *ser*), leukocidins- (*lukF, lukS, lukH, lukD, lukE* and *lukY*), adhesion factors- (belonging to the microbial surface components recognizing adhesive matrix molecules: *clfA, clfB, fnbA, fnbB, fib, map, eno, efb, ebpS, sdrC,* and *sdrE*), and hemolysins- (*hla, hlb, hld, hlgA, hlgB* and *hlgC*) encoding genes. The isolates also harbored the capsule- (*cap8*), the clipase- (*clpB, clpC, clpP, clpX*), the biofilm formation- (*ica* operon), the protease- (*splABCDF*), and the immune evasion cluster- (*sea, sak, chp* and *scn*) encoding genes. Finally, the isolates presented the specialized secretion system Ess (ESAT-6 secretion system) with the *ess* locus, a cluster of eight genes (e.g., *esxAB, essABC, esaABC*). However, these isolates harbored neither exfoliative toxin-encoding genes (*eta, etb, etd*), nor epithelial cell differentiation inhibitors (*edinA, edinB,* and *edinC*), the toxic shock syndrome toxin- (*tst*), and *lukF/S-PV* encoding genes.

For the virulome profile of the *S. aureus* isolated from patient B, the genomic content was similar to isolates from patient A. The differences were the absence of *chp*, the content of enterotoxins-encoding genes (*sea, sed, sej, ser* and *set*) and the presence of the adhesin- (*map*) and the von Willebrand factor-binding protein- (*vWbp*) encoding genes.

2.7. Genetic Basis of Resistance to DAP

A focus on genes involved in DAP resistance was performed. For Patient A, one allelic difference was detected between the two isolates, consisting in one mutation located in MprF protein (L826F) (Figure 1). For Patient B, two allelic differences were noted between the two isolates corresponding to another mutation in MprF protein (S295L) and another one in Cls protein (R228H).

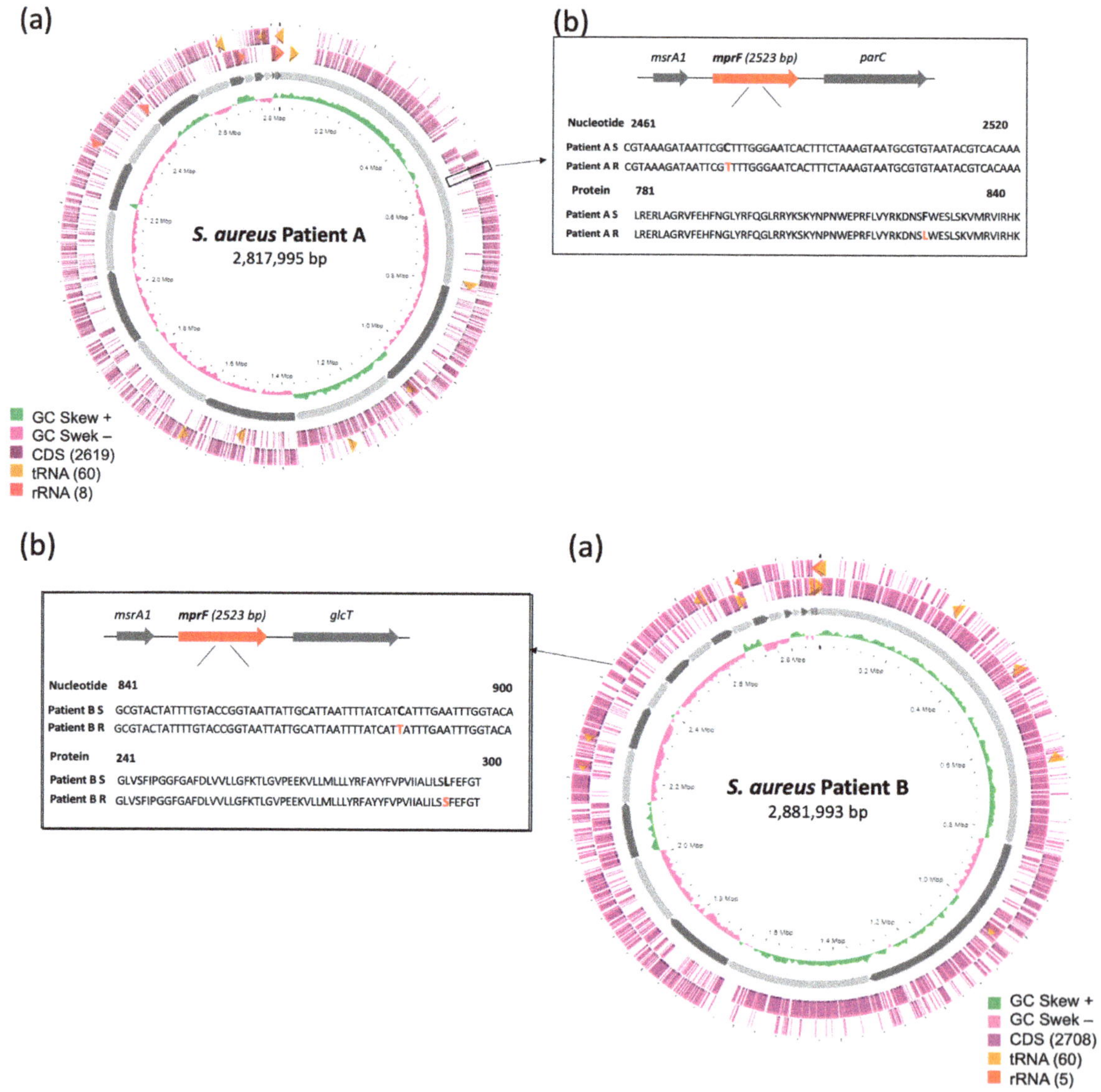

Figure 1. The *mprF* genomic landscape. (**a**) Circular genome representation of patient A and patient B MRSA strains using BRIG software. The inner ring illustrates the GC skew. The outer two rings represent coding sequences (CDS), tRNAs and rRNAs on the reverse and forward strands, respectively. A black box is included to highlight the *mprF* gene. (**b**) Genomic localization of *mprF*. Nucleotide and protein alignments of DAP-susceptible/DAP-resistant isolates from patients A and B, and the mutations detected.

3. Discussion

DAP resistance remains a rare event. Main reports described clinical cases following glycopeptide and DAP therapy [24,27]. In fact, prior exposure to glycopeptides are highlighted as risk factors for decreased susceptibility to DAP [24,28]. These antibiotics induced changes of the bacterial cell wall [28,29]. In this study, we provided two cases of emerging DAP resistance in MRSA during bacteremia, resulting in treatment failure of only

DAP and consequently long-term bacteremia. One of the two patients died when adapted treatment was prescribed, but the link between mortality and the presence of DAP-R strains could not be deduced because this patient approached his end of life. Interestingly, no DAP resistance development was preceded by a modification of VAN susceptibility and no other co-resistance was noted as previously observed [24]. Moreover, it could be observed that DAP was administrated at a well-established dose. However, we cannot evaluate the blood concentration of DAP. There is evidence that a subtherapeutic concentration of this antibiotic favors the development of resistance as previously noted [30].

Globally, the studies on DAP resistance mainly focus on the interaction between the cell membrane and DAP–Ca^{2+} complex [19–26]. The two pairs of isogenic strains showed distinct mutations in the *mprF* gene. The transmembrane MprF protein is responsible for the lysinylation of cell membrane phospholipids and their translocation to the outer leaflet of the cell membrane [31]. This process decreases the negative cell surface charge, leading to the electrostatic repulsion of the cationic anti-microbial peptides such as DAP. Furthermore, this rearrangement has been described as a virulence factor and is widespread in Gram-positive and Gram-negative bacteria [31]. The DAP-R emergence has a fitness cost on the MRSA, with changes in cell wall thickness and cell membrane potential [32]. The MprF protein consists of an N-terminal transmembrane flippase domain, C-terminal catalytic synthase domain, and a central bifunctional domain. The changes in amino acid sequences leading to DAP-R *S. aureus* have been identified in all domains of MprF [33]. S295L mutation was associated with a change in the central bifunctional domain while L826F was related to a change in synthase domain [34]. Cross-resistance to VAN was previously described as associated with *mprF*-mediated DAP-R [35]. Moreover, Capone et al. observed a link between the emergence of in vivo DAP-R *S. aureus* and the glycopeptide therapy [24]. Neither phenomena were observed in our cases; no patients received glycopeptides.

Interestingly, the strain from patient B presented a mutated Cls protein (R228H). A relation between *cls* and DAP resistance has been previously described but exclusively in *Enterococcus* [36,37]. Zhang et al. showed that *cls* gene encoded a cardiolipin synthase, which catalyzed the production of cardiolipin from two molecules of phosphatidylglycerol. The authors suggested that the increase in the concentration of cardiolipin in cell membranes can divert more DAP from its target septum to other sites, thereby improving DAP resistance [9]. The *cls* mutations could modify the distribution of cardiolipins in cell membrane, involving a reduction of these lipids on the cell surface and decreasing the negative charges of membrane cells leading to a reduced adhesion to DAP [37]. We could note that the mutation detected in Cls protein had never been previously described in *Enterococcus* sp. This mutation affected one of phospholipase D-like domains that could alter the catalytic activity of cardiolipin synthase [37]. Investigation on the clear role of the Cls mutation detected in our study and its addition to MprF mutation could be provided in future analysis.

4. Materials and Methods

4.1. Bacterial Identification and Antibiotic Susceptibility Testing

Isolates were identified by mass spectrometry using Vitek® MS system (bioMérieux, Marcy L'Etoile, France) and stored in cryotubes at −80 °C. Antimicrobial susceptibility testing (Penicillin G 1U, cefoxitin 30 µg, erythromycin 15 µg, clindamycin 2 µg, quinupristin-dalfopristin 15 µg, kanamycin 30 µg, tobramycin 10 µg, gentamicin 10 µg, minocycline 30 µg, ofloxacin 5 µg, fusidic acid 10 µg, fosfomycin 200 µg, rifampicin 5 µg, cotrimoxazole 25 µg, linezolid 10 µg) of these isolates was performed by disk diffusion test on Mueller–Hinton (Bio-Rad, Marnes-La-Coquette, France) agar plates according to European Committee for Antimicrobial Susceptibility Testing (EUCAST 2023) recommendations (https://www.eucast.org/clinical_breakpoints accessed on 10 March 2023). Dalbavancin (DAL), ceftaroline (CPT) and ceftobiprole (CBP) MICs were determined by MIC Test Strips (Liofilchem, Roseto degli Abruzzi, Italy and BioMérieux, Marcy l'étoile, France). DAP, VAN and teicoplanin (TEI) MICs were determined using broth microdilution procedures (UMIC)

(Bruker Daltonics, Champs sur Marne, France). Antibiotic susceptibility was interpreted using the EUCAST breakpoints.

4.2. Next-Generation Sequencing

The two pairs of isogenic (DAP-S/DAP-R) *S. aureus* strains were cultivated aerobically at 37 °C for 48 h on Columbia sheep blood agar plates (5%) (BioMérieux). Following the manufacturer's instructions, genomic DNA (gDNA) was extracted from 200 µL of the overnight cultures suspension of the strains using DNeasy UltraClean Microbial Kit (Qiagen, Hilden, Germany) and eluted in 50 µL volume. Quality of gDNA was examined using Qubit fluorometer 2.0 (Invitrogen, Waltham, MA, USA). Whole Genome Sequencing (WGS) was carried out using Illumina MiSeq Sequencing system (Illumina, San Diego, CA, USA). Illumina library preparation was constructed using 250 ng of the extracted DNA following the Nextera XT DNA Prep Kit library paired-end protocol (paired-end read libraries, Illumina) and sequenced in a 39 h run providing 2 × 250 bp reads as previously described [38]. Quality control of the reads was performed directly on MiSeq output reads using FastQC software (v.0.11.7).

4.3. In Silico Analysis

After data quality validation, the *S. aureus* genomes were de novo assembled using Spades software (version 3.15.4) and blasted against the NCBI GenBank database, and also analysed on Type-Strain Genomes Server (https://tygs.dsmz.de/user_requests/new) online platform for more precision in bacteria identification. The first analysis of whole-genome MultiLocus Sequence Typing (wgMLST) was provided using EPISEQ® CS V1-2 software (BioMerieux), a fully integrated web-based software application for genome assemblies and MLST. This software determined the percentage of sequence similarities between two genomes. The finalization of genome annotation was performed using CLC Genomics Workbench software (https://digitalinsights.qiagen.com/products-overview/discovery-insights-portfolio/analysis-and-visualization/qiagen-clc-workbench-premium/?cmpid=QDI_GA_DISC_CLC&gad_source=1&gclid=Cj0KCQiApOyqBhDlARIsAGfnyMqxFp3a-BExOSD0QM3ZwZXsO2JDw4EI5MinfGEm56EPCBijKUwYB_AaArP7EALw_wcB, accessed on 10 March 2023) (Qiagen, Germantown, MA, USA). Pangenome analysis was performed by comparison of the annotated *S. aureus* genomes using Roary tools (Version 3.13.0) available on Galaxy online software (https://www.usegalaxy.org.au/, accessed on 10 March 2023), then visualized on Phandango online tools. ResFinder 4.1, VirulenceFinder 2.0 and PlasmidFinder 2.1 were used for sequence analysis [39–42]. Antimicrobial resistance encoding genes, virulence, pathogenicity, and plasmids were in silico predicted using CGE online platform (http://www.genomicepidemiology.org/services/, accessed on 10 March 2023). Direct comparison between the strains isolated from the same patient was generated using BLAST Ring Image Generator (BRIG) [43]. Single-nucleotide polymorphisms (SNPs) analysis based on whole genome alignment was performed using Snippy [44]. SNP numbers between parental and antibiotic-exposed strains were interpreted according to the criteria of Ankrum and Hall [45], which defined strains with ≤71 SNPs as the "same" strains. All the identified genomics sequences have been deposited on the GenBank website accession bioproject: PRJNA1001284.

5. Conclusions

In conclusion, whilst DAP-R *S. aureus* have been previously described, few papers presented the in vivo acquisition of resistance. These two cases of MRSA isolates became resistant to DAP after around 3 weeks of exposure to this antibiotic. We suggest that *mprF* gene represents a hotspot target to acquire mutations to this antibiotic, particularly in MRSA. A new target has also been described on *cls* gene. This study highlights the non-systematic cross-resistance between DAP and glycopeptides. The use of DAP as first-line therapy at optimal dosages must be considered when patients are at risk of MRSA infection. Moreover, it is crucial to monitor DAP MIC in persistent MRSA bacteremia.

Author Contributions: Conceptualization, A.B.-D., J.-P.L. and A.P.; methodology, A.B.-D. and A.P.; software, C.M. and C.P.; formal analysis, A.B.-D., C.M., C.P. and A.P.; investigation, A.L., F.B., R.L. and A.B.-D.; resources, A.B.-D., C.M., J.-P.L. and A.P.; data curation, A.B.-D., C.M., A.L., C.P., J.-P.L. and A.P.; writing—original draft preparation, A.B.-D., J.-P.L. and A.P.; writing—review and editing, C.M., A.L., C.P., F.B., H.M. and R.L.; visualization, J.-P.L. and A.P.; supervision, H.M. and J.-P.L.; project administration, J.-P.L.; funding acquisition, J.-P.L. All authors have read and agreed to the published version of the manuscript.

Funding: This research received no external funding.

Institutional Review Board Statement: The study was conducted in accordance with the Declaration of Helsinki and approved by the Institutional Review Board of CHU Nîmes (protocol code 6.02.2023, protocol DAP-2023).

Informed Consent Statement: Written informed consent was obtained from the patient B and the patient A's family involved in the study to publish this paper.

Data Availability Statement: All the identified genomics sequences have been deposited on the GenBank website accession bioproject: PRJNA1001284.

Acknowledgments: We thank the Nîmes University hospital for its structural, human and financial support through the award obtained by our team during the internal call for tenders «Thématiques phares». We thank Sarah Kabani for proofreading the manuscript.

Conflicts of Interest: The authors declare no conflict of interest.

References

1. Liu, C.; Bayer, A.; Cosgrove, S.E.; Daum, R.S.; Fridkin, S.K.; Gorwitz, R.J.; Kaplan, S.L.; Karchmer, A.W.; Levine, D.P.; Murray, B.E.; et al. Clinical practice guidelines by the Infectious Diseases Society of America for the treatment of methicillin-resistant *Staphylococcus aureus* infections in adults and children: Executive summary. *Clin. Infect. Dis.* **2011**, *52*, 285–292. [CrossRef] [PubMed]
2. Kaasch, A.J.; Barlow, G.; Edgeworth, J.D.; Fowler, V.G.; Hellmich, M.; Hopkins, S.; Kern, W.V.; Llewelyn, M.J.; Rieg, S.; Rodriguez-Baño, J.; et al. *Staphylococcus aureus* bloodstream infection: A pooled analysis of five prospective, observational studies. *J. Infect.* **2014**, *68*, 242–251. [CrossRef] [PubMed]
3. Fowler, V.G., Jr.; Boucher, H.W.; Corey, G.R.; Abrutyn, E.; Karchmer, A.W.; Rupp, M.E.; Levine, D.P.; Chambers, H.F.; Tally, F.P.; Vigliani, G.A.; et al. *S. aureus* Endocarditis and Bacteremia Study Group. Daptomycin versus standard therapy for bacteremia and endocarditis caused by *Staphylococcus aureus*. *N. Engl. J. Med.* **2006**, *355*, 653–665. [CrossRef] [PubMed]
4. Schweizer, M.L.; Richardson, K.; Vaughan Sarrazin, M.S.; Goto, M.; Livorsi, D.J.; Nair, R.; Alexander, B.; Beck, B.F.; Jones, M.P.; Puig-Asensio, M.; et al. Comparative Effectiveness of Switching to Daptomycin Versus Remaining on Vancomycin Among Patients With Methicillin-resistant *Staphylococcus aureus* (MRSA) Bloodstream Infections. *Clin. Infect. Dis.* **2021**, *72*, S68–S73. [CrossRef] [PubMed]
5. Eisenstein, B.I.; Oleson, F.B., Jr.; Baltz, R.H. Daptomycin: From the mountain to the clinic, with essential help from Francis Tally, MD. *Clin. Infect. Dis.* **2010**, *50*, S10–S15. [CrossRef] [PubMed]
6. Morrisette, T.; Alosaimy, S.; Abdul-Mutakabbir, J.C.; Kebriaei, R.; Rybak, M.J. The Evolving Reduction of Vancomycin and Daptomycin Susceptibility in MRSA-Salvaging the Gold Standards with Combination Therapy. *Antibiotics* **2020**, *9*, 762. [CrossRef]
7. Nguyen, A.H.; Hood, K.S.; Mileykovskaya, E.; Miller, W.R.; Tran, T.T. Bacterial cell membranes and their role in daptomycin resistance: A review. *Front. Mol. Biosci.* **2022**, *9*, 1035574. [CrossRef]
8. Beriashvili, D.; Spencer, N.R.; Dieckmann, T.; Overduin, M.; Palmer, M. Characterization of multimeric daptomycin bound to lipid nanodiscs formed by calcium-tolerant styrene-maleic acid copolymer. *Biochim. Biophys. Acta Biomembr.* **2020**, *1862*, 183234. [CrossRef]
9. Zhang, T.H.; Muraih, J.K.; Tishbi, N.; Herskowitz, J.; Victor, R.L.; Silverman, J.; Uwumarenogie, S.; Taylor, S.D.; Palmer, M.; Mintzer, E. Cardiolipin prevents membrane translocation and permeabilization by daptomycin. *J. Biol. Chem.* **2014**, *289*, 11584–11591. [CrossRef]
10. Silverman, J.A.; Perlmutter, N.G.; Shapiro, H.M. Correlation of daptomycin bactericidal activity and membrane depolarization in *Staphylococcus aureus*. *Antimicrob. Agents Chemother.* **2003**, *47*, 2538–2544. [CrossRef]
11. Fair, R.J.; Tor, Y. Antibiotics and bacterial resistance in the 21st century. *Perspect. Med. Chem.* **2014**, *6*, 25–64. [CrossRef]
12. Foster, T.J. Antibiotic Resistance in *Staphylococcus aureus*. Current Status and Future Prospects. *FEMS Microbiol. Rev.* **2017**, *41*, 430–449. [CrossRef] [PubMed]
13. Sohlenkamp, C.; Geiger, O. Bacterial membrane lipids: Diversity in structures and pathways. *FEMS Microbiol. Rev.* **2016**, *40*, 133–159. [CrossRef] [PubMed]
14. Mengin-Lecreulx, D.; Allen, N.E.; Hobbs, J.N.; van Heijenoort, J. Inhibition of peptidoglycan biosynthesis in *Bacillus* megaterium by daptomycin. *FEMS Microbiol. Lett.* **1990**, *57*, 245–248. [CrossRef] [PubMed]

15. Pogliano, J.; Pogliano, N.; Silverman, J.A. Daptomycin-mediated reorganization of membrane architecture causes mislocalization of essential cell division proteins. *J. Bacteriol.* **2012**, *194*, 4494–4504. [CrossRef]
16. Müller, A.; Wenzel, M.; Strahl, H.; Grein, F.; Saaki, T.N.V.; Kohl, B.; Siersma, T.; Bandow, J.E.; Sahl, H.G.; Schneider, T.; et al. Daptomycin inhibits cell envelope synthesis by interfering with fluid membrane microdomains. *Proc. Natl. Acad. Sci. USA* **2016**, *113*, E7077–E7086. [CrossRef]
17. Grein, F.; Müller, A.; Scherer, K.M.; Liu, X.; Ludwig, K.C.; Klöckner, A.; Strach, M.; Sahl, H.G.; Kubitscheck, U.; Schneider, T. Ca^{2+}-Daptomycin targets cell wall biosynthesis by forming a tripartite complex with undecaprenyl-coupled intermediates and membrane lipids. *Nat. Commun.* **2020**, *11*, 1455. [CrossRef]
18. Kullar, R.; Chin, J.N.; Edwards, D.J.; Parker, D.; Coplin, W.M.; Rybak, M.J. Pharmacokinetics of single-dose daptomycin in patients with suspected or confirmed neurological infections. *Antimicrob. Agents Chemother.* **2011**, *55*, 3505–3509. [CrossRef]
19. Nikolic, P.; Mudgil, P. The Cell Wall, Cell Membrane and Virulence Factors of *Staphylococcus aureus* and Their Role in Antibiotic Resistance. *Microorganisms* **2023**, *11*, 259. [CrossRef]
20. Bayer, A.S.; Schneider, T.; Sahl, H.G. Mechanisms of daptomycin resistance in *Staphylococcus aureus*: Role of the cell membrane and cell wall. *Ann. N. Y. Acad. Sci.* **2013**, *1277*, 139–158. [CrossRef]
21. Miller, W.R.; Bayer, A.S.; Arias, C.A. Mechanism of action and resistance to daptomycin in *Staphylococcus aureus* and enterococci. *Cold Spring Harb. Perspect. Med.* **2016**, *6*, a026997. [CrossRef] [PubMed]
22. Casanova, G.N.; Ruiz, S.M.; Bellido, M.J.L. Mechanisms of Resistance to Daptomycin in *Staphylococcus aureus*. *Rev. Española Quimioter.* **2017**, *30*, 391–396.
23. Tran, T.T.; Munita, J.M.; Arias, C.A. Mechanisms of drug resistance: Daptomycin resistance. *Ann. N. Y. Acad. Sci.* **2015**, *1354*, 32–53. [CrossRef] [PubMed]
24. Capone, A.; Cafiso, V.; Campanile, F.; Parisi, G.; Mariani, B.; Petrosillo, N.; Stefani, S. In vivo development of daptomycin resistance in vancomycin-susceptible methicillin-resistant *Staphylococcus aureus* severe infections previously treated with glycopeptides. *Eur. J. Clin. Microbiol. Infect. Dis.* **2016**, *35*, 625–631. [CrossRef]
25. Bertsche, U.; Yang, S.J.; Kuehner, D.; Wanner, S.; Mishra, N.N.; Roth, T.; Nega, M.; Schneider, A.; Mayer, C.; Grau, T.; et al. Increased cell wall teichoic acid production and D-alanylation are common phenotypes among daptomycin-resistant methicillin-resistant *Staphylococcus aureus* (MRSA) clinical isolates. *PLoS ONE* **2013**, *8*, e67398. [CrossRef]
26. Boyle-Vavra, S.; Jones, M.; Gourley, B.L.; Holmes, M.; Ruf, R.; Balsam, A.R.; Boulware, D.R.; Kline, S.; Jawahir, S.; Devries, A.; et al. Comparative genome sequencing of an isogenic pair of USA800 clinical methicillin-resistant *Staphylococcus aureus* isolates obtained before and after daptomycin treatment failure. *Antimicrob. Agents Chemother.* **2011**, *55*, 2018–2025. [CrossRef] [PubMed]
27. Stefani, S.; Campanile, F.; Santagati, M.; Mezzatesta, M.L.; Cafiso, V.; Pacini, G. Insights and clinical perspectives of daptomycin resistance in *Staphylococcus aureus*: A review of the available evidence. *Int. J. Antimicrob. Agents* **2015**, *46*, 278–289. [CrossRef] [PubMed]
28. Bassetti, M.; Villa, G.; Ansaldi, F.; De Florentiis, D.; Tascini, C.; Cojutti, P.; Righi, E.; Sartor, A.; Crapis, M.; De Rosa, F.G.; et al. Risk factors associated with the onset of daptomycin non-susceptibility in *Staphylococcus aureus* infections in critically ill patients. *Intensive Care Med.* **2015**, *41*, 366–368. [CrossRef]
29. Moise, P.A.; North, D.; Steenbergen, J.N.; Sakoulas, G. Susceptibility relationship between vancomycin and daptomycin in *Staphylococcus aureus*: Facts and assumptions. *Lancet Infect. Dis.* **2009**, *9*, 617–624. [CrossRef] [PubMed]
30. Smirnova, M.V.; Vostrov, S.N.; Strukova, E.V.; Dovzhenko, S.A.; Kobrin, M.B.; Portnoy, Y.A.; Zinner, S.H.; Firsov, A.A. The impact of duration of antibiotic exposure on bacterial resistance predictions using in vitro dynamic models. *J. Antimicrob. Chemother.* **2009**, *64*, 815–820. [CrossRef]
31. Ernst, C.M.; Peschel, A. MprF-mediated daptomycin resistance. *Int. J. Med. Microbiol.* **2019**, *309*, 359–363. [CrossRef] [PubMed]
32. Li, S.; Yin, Y.; Chen, H.; Wang, Q.; Wang, X.; Wang, H. Fitness Cost of Daptomycin-Resistant *Staphylococcus aureus* Obtained from in Vitro Daptomycin Selection Pressure. *Front. Microbiol.* **2017**, *8*, 2199. [CrossRef] [PubMed]
33. Sabat, A.J.; Tinelli, M.; Grundmann, H.; Akkerboom, V.; Monaco, M.; Del Grosso, M.; Errico, G.; Pantosti, A.; Friedrich, A.W. Daptomycin Resistant *Staphylococcus aureus* Clinical Strain With Novel Non-synonymous Mutations in the *mprF* and *vraS* Genes: A New Insight Into Daptomycin Resistance. *Front. Microbiol.* **2018**, *9*, 2705. [CrossRef] [PubMed]
34. Peleg, A.Y.; Miyakis, S.; Ward, D.V.; Earl, A.M.; Rubio, A.; Cameron, D.R.; Pillai, S.; Moellering, R.C., Jr.; Eliopoulos, G.M. Whole genome characterization of the mechanisms of daptomycin resistance in clinical and laboratory derived isolates of *Staphylococcus aureus*. *PLoS ONE* **2012**, *7*, e28316. [CrossRef] [PubMed]
35. Thitiananpakorn, K.; Aiba, Y.; Tan, X.E.; Watanabe, S.; Kiga, K.; Sato'o, Y.; Boonsiri, T.; Li, F.Y.; Sasahara, T.; Taki, Y.; et al. Association of *mprF* mutations with cross-resistance to daptomycin and vancomycin in methicillin-resistant *Staphylococcus aureus* (MRSA). *Sci. Rep.* **2020**, *10*, 16107. [CrossRef] [PubMed]
36. Wang, G.; Yu, F.; Lin, H.; Murugesan, K.; Huang, W.; Hoss, A.G.; Dhand, A.; Lee, L.Y.; Zhuge, J.; Yin, C.; et al. Evolution and mutations predisposing to daptomycin resistance in vancomycin-resistant *Enterococcus faecium* ST736 strains. *PLoS ONE* **2018**, *13*, e0209785. [CrossRef] [PubMed]
37. Li, W.; Hu, J.; Li, L.; Zhang, M.; Cui, Q.; Ma, Y.; Su, H.; Zhang, X.; Xu, H.; Wang, M. New Mutations in *cls* Lead to Daptomycin Resistance in a Clinical Vancomycin- and Daptomycin-Resistant *Enterococcus faecium* Strain. *Front. Microbiol.* **2022**, *13*, 896916. [CrossRef]

38. Pouget, C.; Chatre, C.; Lavigne, J.P.; Pantel, A.; Reynes, J.; Dunyach-Remy, C. Effect of Antibiotic Exposure on *Staphylococcus epidermidis* Responsible for Catheter-Related Bacteremia. *Int. J. Mol. Sci.* **2023**, *24*, 1547. [CrossRef]
39. Carattoli, A.; Zankari, E.; García-Fernández, A.; Voldby Larsen, M.; Lund, O.; Villa, L.; Møller Aarestrup, F.; Hasman, H. In Silico detection and typing of plasmids using PlasmidFinder and plasmid multilocus sequence typing. *Antimicrob. Agents Chemother.* **2014**, *58*, 3895–3903. [CrossRef]
40. Zankari, E.; Allesøe, R.; Joensen, K.G.; Cavaco, L.M.; Lund, O.; Aarestrup, F.M. PointFinder: A novel web tool for WGS-based detection of antimicrobial resistance associated with chromosomal point mutations in bacterial pathogens. *J. Antimicrob. Chemother.* **2017**, *72*, 2764–2768. [CrossRef]
41. Bortolaia, V.; Kaas, R.S.; Ruppe, E.; Roberts, M.C.; Schwarz, S.; Cattoir, V.; Philippon, A.; Allesoe, R.L.; Rebelo, A.R.; Florensa, A.F.; et al. ResFinder 4.0 for Predictions of Phenotypes from Genotypes. *J. Antimicrob. Chemother.* **2020**, *75*, 3491–3500. [CrossRef]
42. Bartels, M.D.; Petersen, A.; Worning, P.; Nielsen, J.B.; Larner-Svensson, H.; Johansen, H.K.; Andersen, L.P.; Jarløv, J.O.; Boye, K.; Larsen, A.R.; et al. Comparing Whole-Genome Sequencing with Sanger Sequencing for Spa Typing of Methicillin-Resistant *Staphylococcus aureus*. *J. Clin. Microbiol.* **2014**, *52*, 4305–4308. [CrossRef]
43. Alikhan, N.F.; Petty, N.K.; Ben Zakour, N.L.; Beatson, S.A. BLAST Ring Image Generator (BRIG): Simple prokaryote genome comparisons. *BMC Genom.* **2011**, *12*, 402. [CrossRef]
44. Snippy: Fast Bacterial Variant Calling from NGS Reads. Available online: https://github.com/tseemann/snippy (accessed on 24 June 2023).
45. Ankrum, A.; Hall, B.G. Population dynamics of *Staphylococcus aureus* in cystic fibrosis patients to determine transmission events by use of whole-genome sequencing. *J. Clin. Microbiol.* **2017**, *55*, 2143–2152. [CrossRef]

antibiotics

MDPI

Article

The Diversity and Zoonotic Potential of *Staphylococcus pseudintermedius* in Humans and Pet Dogs in Trinidad and Tobago

Sharianne Suepaul [1,2,*], Marc Stegger [3,4], Filip Boyen [5], Karla Georges [2] and Patrick Butaye [5,6,7]

1 Department of Pathobiology, School of Veterinary Medicine, St. George's University, True Blue, St. George's FZ818, Grenada
2 Department of Basic Veterinary Sciences, School of Veterinary Medicine, Faculty of Medical Sciences, The University of the West Indies, St. Augustine 685509, Trinidad and Tobago; karla.georges@sta.uwi.edu
3 Department of Bacteria, Parasites, and Fungi, Statens Serum Institut, 2300 Copenhagen, Denmark; mtg@ssi.dk
4 Antimicrobial Resistance and Infectious Diseases Laboratory, Harry Butler Institute, Murdoch University, Perth, WA 6150, Australia
5 Department of Pathobiology, Pharmacology and Wildlife Medicine, Faculty of Veterinary Medicine, Ghent University, 9820 Merelbeke, Belgium; filip.boyen@ugent.be (F.B.); patrick.butaye@ugent.be or pabutaye@cityu.edu.hk (P.B.)
6 Department of Infectious Diseases and Public Health, Jockey Club College of Veterinary Medicine and Life Sciences, City University of Hong Kong, Kowloon, Hong Kong
7 School of Veterinary Medicine, Ross University, Basseterre P.O. Box 334, Saint Kitts and Nevis
* Correspondence: ssuepaul@sgu.edu

Abstract: *Staphylococcus pseudintermedius* is an opportunistic pathogen that is frequently isolated from canines. It is of escalating interest because of its increasing antimicrobial resistance and zoonotic potential. Although many published articles are available that describe isolates obtained from diseased dogs and humans, this study focused on isolates obtained from healthy dogs and their owners who presented at clinics for routine veterinary care and utilized whole genome sequencing-based analyses for strain comparisons. A total of 25 humans and 27 canines were sampled at multiple sites, yielding 47 and 45 isolates, respectively. Whole genome sequence analysis was performed. We detected mostly new sequence types (STs) and a high diversity. Strains carried few antimicrobial resistance genes and plasmids, albeit three MRSP strains were found that belonged to two internationally distributed STs. The virulence content did not provide insights toward a tendency to colonization of humans but supported that there may be differences in the surface proteins between carrier strains and those causing pyoderma. We identified 13 cases in which humans were infected with strains from the dog they owned.

Keywords: *Staphylococcus pseudintermedius*; methicillin-resistant; diversity; virulence; dog; human; comparative genomics

1. Introduction

Staphylococci are opportunistic organisms that can cause infections in humans and animals [1]. This genus is mainly investigated for its molecular epidemiology, virulence [2,3], and antimicrobial resistance [4,5]. The current study focused on *Staphylococcus pseudintermedius*, which commonly causes pyogenic soft tissue infections, otitis externa, sinusitis, osteomyelitis, endocarditis, and post-operative abscesses [6–8]. *S. pseudintermedius* regularly colonizes dogs and cats at multiple sites such as the skin and mucous membranes [9,10] but may also be isolated from horses [11] and humans [12].

Dogs are of particular interest since up to 90% of dogs have been shown to carry this bacterium [13]. Additionally, different strains of *S. pseudintermedius* can inhabit different sites of a dog at the same time, which has vast implications for diagnostic testing and the determination of antimicrobial sensitivity [14]. This organism can be zoonotic because it can be transferred from pet dogs to their human owners, and there is the potential for *S. pseudintermedius* to cause infections in humans, particularly in immunocompromised individuals [15]. Although carriage of *S. pseudintermedius* may be short-term and sporadic in healthy humans, dogs can be carriers for extended periods of time [13].

Antimicrobial resistance in *S. pseudintermedius* is of growing concern, especially the methicillin-resistant *S. pseudintermedius* (MRSP) strains [16–19]. Like methicillin-resistant *Staphylococcus aureus* (MRSA), MRSP has evolved via the horizontal transfer, acquisition, and insertion of the staphylococcal cassette chromosome (SCC), which carries a *mec* gene (*mecA* or C) as well as other genes encoding virulence characteristics, other resistance genes, and metal resistances [20]. The *mecA* gene encodes an alternative penicillin-binding protein (PBP2a) that has a low affinity for β-lactam antibiotics [21], leading to resistance to these commonly used antibiotics. MRSP strains have also been associated with resistance to multiple classes of antimicrobials and hence are termed multidrug-resistant (MDR). The occurrence of these antimicrobial-resistant strains is unsettling because it limits the options for therapeutic management of infections and has a grave impact on morbidity and mortality [6].

Recently, there has been increasing evidence of the role of MRSP in causing infections in canines as well as humans [22], including the transmission of *Staphylococcus pseudintermedius* between humans [23,24]. This is mainly due to the advancement in the techniques used to identify the *Staphylococcus* species, which include matrix-assisted laser desorption/ionization–time of flight (MALDI-TOF) mass spectrometry and the combination of molecular subtyping and sequencing techniques that aid in increasing the accuracy of identifying *S. pseudintermedius* infections [13]. As a result, there is a rapidly growing pool of genomic data available regarding *S. pseudintermedius*. Most of the data involve MRSP, which displays a rather a clonal population structure [4]. Although there are many different sequence types, a geographical pattern of distribution was observed by Perreten et al. in 2010 [25], when ST71 was the major clone observed in Europe and ST68 was the major clone observed in the USA. Recent studies published in 2022 indicated that ST71 is currently the major MRSP clone observed globally [4,26,27].

There is an increasing interest in identifying and comparing the various virulence factors and colonization capacities possessed by the various sequence types of both MRSP and methicillin-susceptible *S. pseudintermedius* (MSSP) to determine if there are any associations with in vivo virulence. Thus far, there are indications that the surface proteins (*spsD/F/P/Q*) that are involved in colonization might be predominant in those isolates that cause pyoderma in dogs [28], indicating that these isolates may exhibit a higher pathogenicity. The genes encoding for *spsL* and *spsD* have been associated with host specificity; however, further research is required for confirmation because these genes show a high sequence variation [29].

The objectives of this study were to elucidate the clonal types of *S. pseudintermedius* present in Trinidad and Tobago and to determine the zoonotic potential and specific characteristics of the accessory genome of strains isolated from healthy dogs and their owners using genome sequencing.

2. Results

2.1. Strains

Seventy-two strains were included in this study. They originated from 27 apparently healthy dogs and 25 owners of these dogs, representing 25 human–dog pairs and 2 dogs for which their owner was negative. Forty-five strains originated from dogs, and twenty-seven were from humans. Of the dog strains, 17 were isolated from the nose, 18 were from the mouth, and 10 were from the skin of the abdomen. Of the human strains, 8 were isolated from the nose, 5 were from the mouth, and 14 were from the hands (Table 1).

2.2. MLST

Only seven previously identified STs (ST1709, ST1097, ST373, ST758, ST71, ST45, and ST192) representing 12 strains were found amongst the 72 strains. All other isolates presented novel sequence types, as shown in Figure 1. One strain could not be typed due to absence of the *pta* gene. An eBURST analysis demonstrated that the strains were singletons.

Table 1. Origin of the strains investigated.

Animal	Number of Isolates	Isolation Site		
		Nose (n)	Mouth (n)	Abdomen (Dog) Hand (Human) (n)
Dog (n = 27)	45	17	18	10
Human (n = 25)	27	8	5	14

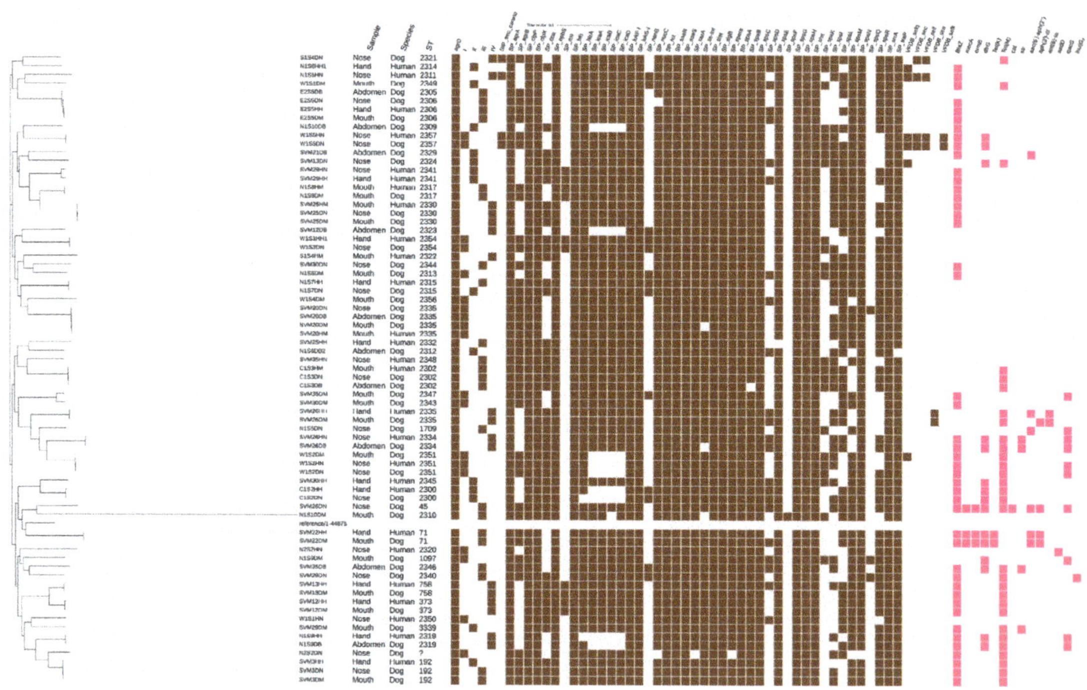

Figure 1. SNP-based phylogenetic tree and accessory genome of the analyzed *S. pseudintermedius* strains. New sequence types all had STs higher than 2300. Virulence genes are shown in brown, and resistance genes are all in purple. Samples are named according to their origin; the last letters signify whether the strain originated from a dog (D) or human (H) sampling site with N for nose, H for hand, B for abdomenal skin, and M for mouth. Strains with the same prefix were from the same dog–owner combination. The strain named reference 1-44876 was the *S. pseudintermedius* reference genome ATCC 49051.

2.3. Phylogeny

In all cases, not a single dog–human combination contained exactly the same strain, with all showing at least one SNP difference (Table S1 in the Supplementary Materials). In 13 cases, the SNP differences were between 1 and 12, indicating that both isolates represented the same clone or strain. A second group of two cases could be identified with the number of SNPs between 12 and 50, and finally a third group with more than 50 SNPs included nine cases. In the latter group, no transfer of the strain could be demonstrated, while in the second group, it was unclear whether these strains represented the same clone and transmission had occurred. However, multiple strains colonizing the same dog (as well as multiple strains in a human in a few cases) were observed. In one dog, two identical strains were isolated from different sampling sites (Figure 1).

We isolated *S. pseudintermedius* at multiple sites on dogs (nose, mouth, and ventral abdomen) and obtained several isolates from the same dog. We obtained multiple strains (two to four strains) from 15 dogs; in 5 of the cases the isolates represented the same strain (less than 12 SNPs), and in 10 cases, the isolates were different strains.

In contrast, although we sampled multiple anatomical sites in humans (nose, mouth and hands), we isolated significantly (chi-squared; $p = 0.008$) fewer strains from different sites from a single human than from dogs. We obtained two isolates from five people, and in four of those cases, the isolates represented different strains (more than 12 SNPs). In one single case, the same strain was isolated twice.

2.4. Antimicrobial Resistance (AMR) Genes

It is important to note that the isolates utilized in this study were not independent because we isolated them from owners and dogs in the same household as well as multiple clones from one dog. As such, there was a bias in the dataset for duplicates. Seventeen strains were fully susceptible, and a few strains carried multiple resistance genes. Forty-five out of seventy-two strains carried a *blaZ*, and three MRSPs were identified: two ST71s from a dog and his owner and one ST45 from the nose of a dog. The *mecA* gene in the ST71 strain was located in the SCC*mec* type III(3A), while the SCC*mec* element of the ST45 strain was non-typeable as commonly noted in CC45 strains [25]. A BLASTN analysis of the formerly described non-categorized $\psi SCCmec_{57395}$ revealed a 100% identity with this element; when using easyfig [30], the structure was shown to be the same. Thirty strains were *tet*(M)-positive, and two strains (the MRSP ST72) carried the *tet*(K) gene. Fifteen strains carried the *dfrG* gene. All other AMR genes were only carried by between one and six strains. Resistance to quaternary ammonium compounds mediated by the *qacG* gene was carried by ten strains (Figure 1).

2.5. Plasmids

Few strains carried plasmids, and even fewer carried more than one. A total of 17 strains carried one or more plasmid replicons. One strain carried two plasmids, and the MRSP strain ST45 carried four plasmids. The most common plasmid replicon found was the repUS43 replicon, which was carried by 15 strains. The second most common was the rep7a replicon, which was carried by four strains, of which two also carried the repUS43 replicon. The additional replicons found (repUS12 and rep13) were carried by the ST45 MRSP that also carried the other two replicons.

2.6. Virulence Genes

S. pseudintermedius virulence genes were found in all strains (Figure 1). Using the VFDBins, only a few enterotoxins (*sea*, *sec*, *selI*, *selK*, and *selq*) were found in a few strains. Using the *S. pseudintermedius* database to compare these strains, it was found that all strains contained the enterotoxin-encoding genes (*seaR* and *seaS*), all but three contained the *se-int*, and only few contained the *sec-canine*. The accessory gene regulator genes (*agrA* and *agrD*) were found in all strains, while the *agrB* gene was frequently absent. All four described types of *agrD* were detected. The most common type was type III with 22 strains that were positive. Types I and IV were found in 17 strains, and type II was found in 14 strains. Other virulence gene regulators present in all strains were the global regulator (*rot*, *srrA*, and *sigB*), and the *traP* and *sarA* genes were detected in all but one strain. All strains also contained genes encoding leukotoxins (lukF-I and lukS-I), proteases (*clpP* and *clpX*), the elastin binding protein gene (*ebpS*), β-hemolysin (*hlb*), and all but one surface protease (*htrA*). While all strains contained the exfoliative toxin gene (*siet*), all but one contained the *speta* gene, few contained the exfoliative toxin genes *exi* (10) and *expB* (9), and none the *expA* gene. Most of the strains had the capacity to form biofilms since they contained the *icaA/B/C/D* genes (63/72). All but two strains contained the nuclease gen *nucC*, and slightly more than half contained the coagulase gene *coa*. The sialidase encoding gene *nanB* was found in 13 strains. Several staphylococcal surface proteins were present, of which some were in all strains while others were in fewer strains. The *spsJ*, *spsO*, and *spsP* genes were not detected.

2.7. Prophages

All strains carried prophages, of which some were only incomplete phages. Due to the multitude of incomplete phages, it was not possible to make concise comparisons. However, similar-sized phages were found in the dog–owner pairs as well as similar sizes of incomplete phages. There was certainly a great variety of different sizes of prophages amongst the strains within the same ST and between the different STs.

3. Discussion

In contrast to most other studies that focused on MRSP, we sequenced a collection of colonizing strains that included the strains that also infected the owner of the dog. To our knowledge, there is only one study that used WGS and thus unambiguously showed transmission [23]. We studied apparently healthy animals that came to veterinary clinics for routine checkups or vaccinations.

3.1. Genetic Diversity

Most of the strains represented new STs and were singletons indicating a geographically specific population structure of *S. pseudintermedius* in Trinidad. New STs of *S. pseudintermedius* from dogs have been frequently reported in as yet underexplored regions [27,31,32], and these studies showed a specific geographical association of *S. pseudintermedius* sequence types. In contrast, MRSP isolates were more common STs with the European MRSP ST71, which was identified in one dog–human pair, and the MRSP ST45, which was only found in a dog. This study detected the most reported MRSP clones (ST71 and ST45 [33]), indicating a worldwide expansion of these clones that includes the Caribbean region, probably through tourism or animal trade. While the US is geographically closer, the MRSP ST68 clone, which is typically associated with the US [33], was not detected. Nevertheless, in Trinidad, MRSP does not seem to be highly prevalent because most strains are MSSP.

The MRSP ST71 was also found on an owner, while the MRSP ST45 strain was not found on an owner. There were no real indications that there was a difference in colonization capacity between the two detected MRSP clones because we did not detect any difference in the virulence genes apart from the *coa* and *spsI* genes, which were present in the ST45 strain but not in the ST71 strain. Intriguingly, the human ST71 strain, while being nearly identical (only one SNP difference) in all investigated accessory genes, lacked the *spsD* gene. Whether this was associated with an adaptation after colonization of the owner remains to be determined.

One strain could not be typed using MLST because the *pta* gene was absent. The *pta* gene encodes a phosphate acetyltransferase, and to the best of our knowledge, the absence of that gene has never been reported previously. Assuming that the gene was incompletely sequenced, we were not able to locate potential parts of the gene in the sequence. Upon observation of the cluster pattern of the strain (N2S2DN; Figure 1), it was observed that it was not clustering together with a specific sequence type. Thus, we assumed that this gene was absent in this strain and that this was a rare finding.

It has been shown previously using different methods that the genetic diversity of strains in a single individual dog can be considerable [34]. Also, in our study, this was evident, although there were also quite a number of dogs with the same clone present. This was less obvious in humans, although it should be noted that there were also fewer humans from whom we could obtain multiple isolates using our methodology. We did not find any indication that certain *S. pseudintermedius* strains colonize humans better than animals.

Transmission of *S. pseudintermedius* from dogs to humans has been studied on several occasions [29,35]. The transfer, which has been demonstrated at different degrees, is also dependent on the sampling methods used as well as whether the dog was experiencing pyoderma, making it difficult to estimate transmission rates in general. The same/similar strains have been found to colonize both the animal and the owner, though colonization with unrelated strains has also been demonstrated [24,36,37]. High diversity may account for the variation amongst strains colonizing dogs and humans. Indeed, it has been shown that there was a large diversity of strains on the same dog and that the detection of types differed over time [38]. As such, the absence of the strain that was found on the owner and dog may be merely a result of this high diversity of strains and the limited number of isolates investigated from each dog in this study. A study assessing the diversity of strains from the same dog would be of interest.

3.2. *AMR*

In this study, only 3 out of 72 strains were methicillin-resistant, and the other strains were broadly susceptible to most antibiotics. The resistance against antimicrobials in *S. pseudintermedius* is quite variable according to the studies performed, though MRSP strains tend to be increasingly prevalent, and those strains tend to be multidrug-resistant [39, 40], as also seen in our study. The AMR genes found in these strains are the classical resistance genes often found in *S. pseudintermedius* [41,42].

3.3. *Plasmids*

Though the resistance genes detected are frequently associated with plasmids [42], few plasmids were present, and most of the strains were devoid of plasmids. The repUS43 replicon has been found in different Gram-positive bacteria worldwide (assessed through a BLAST search of the sequence and has been shown to be associated with plasmids carrying the antimicrobial resistance gene, although in our study, no such association could be found, which may have been caused by the fact that the assembly did not allow for a closed sequence. Typically, the MRSP strains carried the rep7a, and only one MSSP carried a plasmid with this replicon; this replicon also has been found in a multitude of Gram-positive bacteria (via BLAST search). The MRSP ST45 carried most plasmids with all four different replicons we detected.

3.4. *Virulence*

The *S. pseudintermedius* strains isolated in this study seemed to have a core virulence gene content similar to previously studied strains [43]. Four genes coding for surface proteins (*spsD*, *spsF*, *spsP*, and *spsQ*) involved in colonization by binding to the host's extracellular matrix were previously shown to be present mainly in dog pyoderma isolates [28], although this was not absolute. In our collection of strains, we detected these genes to a lesser extent than most of the other surface proteins (23, 1, 0, and 3, respectively). It is striking that three of those surface proteins were nearly absent, indicating that those genes may indeed be of importance in pyoderma since our strains were from healthy dogs. This indicated that the strains used in this study were mainly the typical colonizing strains and that these strains can readily colonize humans.

Differences in virulence and phage content have been found between human and dog MRSP strains of a same ST, including an ST45 strain [44] similar to that in our study. On the other hand, in a larger collection of strains, no differences could be found [29]. Unfortunately, the owner of the dog carrying this ST45 strain did not carry the same strain. The ST71 strain of our study showed a difference with the human strain lacking the *spsD* gene, while in the study by Phumthanakor et al. (2021) [44], the *spsP* and *spsQ* genes were differently present in the dog and human strains. Nevertheless, these surface proteins are probably associated with pyoderma in dogs. It may thus well be that these proteins were lost since they are specific for adhesion to dog keratinocytes. Differences were also seen in the phages; however, since our sequences were Illumina-generated sequences, the comparison of the presence of phages was not possible. Though several differences were noted, they might have been artificial because they were partially located on different contigs. Long-read sequencing could solve this issue.

Other differences were noted between strains of the same ST, and those were mainly seen in different surface proteins (*spsB/D/I/L/Q/R*). Other genes that differed were the enterotoxin *se-int* and the nuclease *nunC*. Differences in the presence was also seen for several *sps* genes within a sequence type, which has been noted before [43]. The reason why these surface proteins differ so much between clonally related strains compared to other genes remains to be elucidated.

4. Materials and Methods

4.1. Isolates

The isolates were obtained from dogs and their owners and identified using MALDI-TOF in a previous study [45]. Sampling in this former study was done on dog–owner combinations with the aim to isolate all Staphylococcaceae and determine the species distribution and overlaps as well as the antimicrobial susceptibility of the isolates. The *S. pseudintermedius* isolates included in this study were selected from this collection based on the presence of an isolate in a dog and owner. From several dogs and owners, several isolates were obtained from different locations and subsequently subjected to genome sequencing. There were isolates included from two dogs for which the owner isolate was excluded because of contamination of the DNA sample that became evident after sequence analysis.

4.2. Whole Genome Sequencing and Sequence Analysis

Overnight cultures were grown in tryptic soy broth at 37 °C with 200 rpm shaking. Genomic DNA was extracted using the DNeasy Blood and Tissue kit (Qiagen). Library preparation was carried out using the Nextera XT kit and paired-end 2 × 250 nbp sequencing on a MiSeq, all following standard Illumina protocols (Illumina Inc., San Diego, CA, USA). All raw reads were deposited under bioproject PRJNA778212 (BioSamples: SAMN22933514 and SAMN31370566-SAMN31370626).

De novo assembly was conducted using a unicycler, quality was assessed with QUAST, and sequences were annotated using RASTk on the Patric server (https://www.patricbrc.org/ accessed on 6 August 2022). MLST was performed on the CGE server using 'MLST' (https://cge.cbs.dtu.dk/services/MLST/, accessed for this manuscript on 12 August 2022) [46]. Unknown MLST profiles and alleles were submitted to the 'Public databases for molecular typing and microbial genome diversity' (https://pubmlst.org/ accessed for this manuscript on 2 November 2022), and new allele numbers and sequence types were obtained. MLST profiles were compared using BURST on pubMLST.

To investigate the genetic relatedness of the isolates, we used CSI Phylogeny 1.4 on the CGE server (http://www.genomicepidemiology.org/ accessed for this manuscript on 20 August 2022) for SNP analysis [47] using the *S. pseudintermedius* reference genome ATCC 49051 (named 1-44876). The relatedness of the isolates was visualized using ITol [48].

The following analyses were performed with pipelines from the Center for Genomic Epidemiology (http://www.genomicepidemiology.org/ accessed for this manuscript on 25 August 20222): Kmer analysis to confirm the species identification (KmerFinder) [49], ResFinder v.3.0 for the detection of resistance genes [50], PlasmidFinder v2.0 for the detection of plasmid replicons [51], and SCC*mec*Finder for identification of the SCC*mec* type. Sequences not included in the SCC*mec* typing scheme were downloaded, and BLASTN was used for finding similar sequences. Structure of the pseudoSCC*mec* elements was compared using easyfig [30]. Phages were analyzed using Phaster (https://phaster.ca/ accessed for this manuscript on 27 October 2022) [52].

Virulence genes were determined with Abricate using vfdb [53] and a database specifically developed for the detection of *S. pseudintermedius* virulence genes (DB_SP) [43]. The specific database contained the sequences for *spsA-R*, *clpP*, *siet*, *speta*, *se-int*, *lukF-I*, *lukS-I*, *sec-canine*, *exi*, *expB*, *agrA-D*, *icaA-D*, *nanB*, *coa*, *clpX*, *saeR*, *saeS*, *htrA*, *nucC*, *hlb*, *sigB*, *srrA*, *sarA*, *rot*, *traP*, *expA*, and *epbS*. We determined the four different *agrD* types (GenBank accession nos. EU157356.1, EU157391.1, EU157400.1, and EU157402.1) using BLASTN on the Patric server [34].

Statistical analysis of differences between prevalence of characteristics between dogs and humans were assessed via the chi-squared test.

5. Conclusions

Less than half of the sampled dog–owner combinations showed that humans were colonized with *S. pseudintermedius* strains of the healthy dog they owned (defined as less than 12 SNPs). In some cases, other strains were found, although this may merely have reflected the high diversity of *S. pseudintermedius* strains that can be present within one dog. We identified mostly new STs and a high diversity of *S. pseudintermedius* strains in Trinidad. Strains carried few antimicrobial resistance genes and few plasmids, albeit three MRSP strains were found belonging to two internationally distributed STs. There were no indications that strains isolated from owners possessed specific virulence genes that could facilitate the colonization of humans.

Supplementary Materials: The following supporting information can be downloaded at https://www.mdpi.com/article/10.3390/antibiotics12081266/s1, Table S1. SNP Matrix.

Author Contributions: Conceptualization, P.B. and S.S.; methodology, P.B., F.B. and M.S.; validation, all authors; formal analysis, P.B.; resources, P.B. and S.S.; data curation, P.B.; writing—original draft preparation, P.B. and S.S.; writing—review and editing, all authors; visualization, P.B.; supervision, P.B.; project administration, P.B.; funding acquisition, P.B. and S.S. All authors have read and agreed to the published version of the manuscript.

Funding: This research was funded by the University of the West Indies Campus Research and Publication Fund (grant number CRP.3.MAR16.36), the Ross University School of Veterinary Medicine (grant number 22/001) and The MALDI-TOF MS was financed by the Research Foundation Flanders (FWO-Vlaanderen) as a Hercules project [G0H2516N, AUGE/15/05].

Institutional Review Board Statement: Ethical approval was obtained from the University of the West Indies Ethics Committee (reference number CEC227/06/16).

Informed Consent Statement: Witnessed verbal informed consent was obtained from all owners for sample collection. No minors were sampled during this study.

Data Availability Statement: The raw sequence data are available from the NCBI under BioProject PRJNA892162, BioSample SAMN22933514, and SRA numbers SRR21977355 to SRR21977426.

Acknowledgments: We are grateful to Tesha Sooklal and Nirvana Mahabir for their assistance in the DNA extraction and quantification process. We thank Serge Verbanck for his skillful technical assistance during the MALDI-TOF analyses.

Conflicts of Interest: The authors declare no conflict of interest.

References

1. Fàbregas, N.; Pérez, D.; Viñes, J.; Cuscó, A.; Migura-García, L.; Ferrer, L.; Francino, O. Diverse Populations of *Staphylococcus pseudintermedius* Colonize the Skin of Healthy Dogs. *Microbiol. Spectr.* **2023**, *11*, e0339322. [CrossRef]
2. Cengiz, S.; Okur, S.; Oz, C.; Turgut, F.; Gumurcinler, B.; Sevuk, N.S.; Kekec, A.I.; Cepoglu, H.; Sevimli, U.; Adiguzel, M.C. Prevalence and clonal diversity of methicillin-resistant *Staphylococcus aureus* and methicillin-resistant *Staphylococcus pseudintermedius* isolated from dogs and cats with eye discharge. *Acta Microbiol. Immunol. Hung.* **2023**, *70*, 134–141. [CrossRef]
3. Fàbregas, N.; Pérez, D.; Viñes, J.; Fonticoba, R.; Cuscó, A.; Migura-García, L.; Ferrer, L.; Francino, O. Whole-Genome Sequencing and De Novo Assembly of 67 *Staphylococcus pseudintermedius* Strains Isolated from the Skin of Healthy Dogs. *Microbiol. Resour. Announc.* **2022**, *11*, e0003922. [CrossRef]

4. Adiguzel, M.C.; Schaefer, K.; Rodriguez, T.; Ortiz, J.; Sahin, O. Prevalence, Mechanism, Genetic Diversity, and Cross-Resistance Patterns of Methicillin-Resistant *Staphylococcus* Isolated from Companion Animal Clinical Samples Submitted to a Veterinary Diagnostic Laboratory in the Midwestern United States. *Antibiotics* **2022**, *11*, 609. [CrossRef]
5. Glajzner, P.; Szewczyk, E.M.; Szemraj, M. Pathogenic potential and antimicrobial resistance of *Staphylococcus pseudintermedius* isolated from human and animals. *Folia Microbiol.* **2022**, *68*, 231–243. [CrossRef]
6. Costa, S.S.; Ribeiro, R.; Serrano, M.; Oliveira, K.; Ferreira, C.; Leal, M.; Pomba, C.; Couto, I. *Staphylococcus aureus* Causing Skin and Soft Tissue Infections in Companion Animals: Antimicrobial Resistance Profiles and Clonal Lineages. *Antibiotics* **2022**, *11*, 599. [CrossRef]
7. Gagetti, P.; Wattam, A.R.; Giacoboni, G.; De Paulis, A.; Bertona, E.; Corso, A.; Rosato, A.E. Identification and molecular epidemiology of methicillin resistant *Staphylococcus pseudintermedius* strains isolated from canine clinical samples in Argentina. *BMC Vet. Res.* **2019**, *15*, 264. [CrossRef] [PubMed]
8. Silva, V.; Oliveira, A.; Manageiro, V.; Caniça, M.; Contente, D.; Capita, R.; Alonso-Calleja, C.; Carvalho, I.; Capelo, J.L.; Igrejas, G.; et al. Clonal Diversity and Antimicrobial Resistance of Methicillin-Resistant *Staphylococcus pseudintermedius* Isolated from Canine Pyoderma. *Microorganisms* **2021**, *9*, 482. [CrossRef] [PubMed]
9. Bierowiec, K.; Miszczak, M.; Korzeniowska-Kowal, A.; Wzorek, A.; Płókarz, D.; Gamian, A. Epidemiology of *Staphylococcus pseudintermedius* in cats in Poland. *Sci. Rep.* **2021**, *11*, 18898. [CrossRef] [PubMed]
10. Dazio, V.; Nigg, A.; Schmidt, J.S.; Brilhante, M.; Campos-Madueno, E.I.; Mauri, N.; Kuster, S.P.; Brawand, S.G.; Willi, B.; Endimiani, A.; et al. Duration of carriage of multidrug-resistant bacteria in dogs and cats in veterinary care and co-carriage with their owners. *One Health* **2021**, *13*, 100322. [CrossRef]
11. De Martino, L.; Lucido, M.; Mallardo, K.; Facello, B.; Mallardo, M.; Iovane, G.; Pagnini, U.; Tufano, M.A.; Catalanotti, P. Methicillin-resistant staphylococci isolated from healthy horses and horse personnel in Italy. *J. Vet. Diagn. Invest.* **2010**, *22*, 77–82. [CrossRef]
12. Latronico, F.; Moodley, A.; Nielsen, S.S.; Guardabassi, L. Enhanced adherence of methicillin-resistant *Staphylococcus pseudintermedius* sequence type 71 to canine and human corneocytes. *Vet. Res.* **2014**, *45*, 70. [CrossRef] [PubMed]
13. Somayaji, R.; Rubin, J.E.; Priyantha, M.A.; Church, D. Exploring *Staphylococcus pseudintermedius*: An emerging zoonotic pathogen? *Future Microbiol.* **2016**, *11*, 1371–1374. [CrossRef]
14. Frosini, S.M.; Bond, R.; King, R.H.; Loeffler, A. The nose is not enough: Multi-site sampling is best for MRSP detection in dogs and households. *Vet. Dermatol.* **2022**, *33*, 576–580. [CrossRef] [PubMed]
15. Wegener, A.; Duim, B.; van der Graaf-van Bloois, L.; Zomer, A.L.; Visser, C.E.; Spaninks, M.; Timmerman, A.J.; Wagenaar, J.A.; Broens, E.M. Within-Household Transmission and Bacterial Diversity of *Staphylococcus pseudintermedius*. *Pathogens* **2022**, *11*, 850. [CrossRef] [PubMed]
16. Bardasheva, A.; Tikunov, A.; Kozlova, Y.; Zhirakovskaia, E.; Fedorets, V.; Fomenko, N.; Kalymbetova, T.; Chretien, S.; Pavlov, V.; Tikunova, N.; et al. Antibiotic Resistance and Pathogenomics of Staphylococci Circulating in Novosibirsk, Russia. *Microorganisms* **2021**, *9*, 2487. [CrossRef] [PubMed]
17. Jantorn, P.; Heemmamad, H.; Soimala, T.; Indoung, S.; Saising, J.; Chokpaisarn, J.; Wanna, W.; Tipmanee, V.; Saeloh, D. Antibiotic Resistance Profile and Biofilm Production of *Staphylococcus pseudintermedius* Isolated from Dogs in Thailand. *Pharmaceuticals* **2021**, *14*, 592. [CrossRef] [PubMed]
18. Kang, J.H.; Chung, T.H.; Hwang, C.Y. Clonal distribution of methicillin-resistant *Staphylococcus pseudintermedius* isolates from skin infection of dogs in Korea. *Vet. Microbiol.* **2017**, *210*, 32–37. [CrossRef]
19. Menandro, M.L.; Dotto, G.; Mondin, A.; Martini, M.; Ceglie, L.; Pasotto, D. Prevalence and characterization of methicillin-resistant *Staphylococcus pseudintermedius* from symptomatic companion animals in Northern Italy: Clonal diversity and novel sequence types. *Comp. Immunol. Microbiol. Infect. Dis.* **2019**, *66*, 101331. [CrossRef]
20. Gan, T.; Shu, G.; Fu, H.; Yan, Q.; Zhang, W.; Tang, H.; Yin, L.; Zhao, L.; Lin, J. Antimicrobial resistance and genotyping of *Staphylococcus aureus* obtained from food animals in Sichuan Province, China. *BMC Vet. Res.* **2021**, *17*, 177. [CrossRef]
21. Moses, I.B.; Santos, F.F.; Gales, A.C. Human Colonization and Infection by *Staphylococcus pseudintermedius*: An Emerging and Underestimated Zoonotic Pathogen. *Microorganisms* **2023**, *11*, 581. [CrossRef]
22. Afshar, M.F.; Zakaria, Z.; Cheng, C.H.; Ahmad, N.I. Prevalence and multidrug-resistant profile of methicillin-resistant *Staphylococcus aureus* and methicillin-resistant *Staphylococcus pseudintermedius* in dogs, cats, and pet owners in Malaysia. *Vet. World* **2023**, *16*, 536–545. [CrossRef] [PubMed]
23. Abdullahi, I.N.; Lozano, C.; Zarazaga, M.; Saidenberg, A.B.S.; Stegger, M.; Torres, C. Clonal relatedness of coagulase-positive staphylococci among healthy dogs and dog-owners in Spain. Detection of multidrug-resistant-MSSA-CC398 and novel linezolid-resistant-MRSA-CC5. *Front. Microbiol.* **2023**, *14*, 1121564. [CrossRef] [PubMed]
24. Cuny, C.; Layer-Nicolaou, F.; Weber, R.; Köck, R.; Witte, W. Colonization of Dogs and Their Owners with *Staphylococcus aureus* and *Staphylococcus pseudintermedius* in Households, Veterinary Practices, and Healthcare Facilities. *Microorganisms* **2022**, *10*, 677. [CrossRef] [PubMed]
25. Perreten, V.; Kadlec, K.; Schwarz, S.; Grönlund Andersson, U.; Finn, M.; Greko, C.; Moodley, A.; Kania, S.A.; Frank, L.A.; Bemis, D.A.; et al. Clonal spread of methicillin-resistant *Staphylococcus pseudintermedius* in Europe and North America: An international multicentre study. *J. Antimicrob. Chemother.* **2010**, *65*, 1145–1154. [CrossRef] [PubMed]

26. Bruce, S.A.; Smith, J.T.; Mydosh, J.L.; Ball, J.; Needle, D.B.; Gibson, R.; Andam, C.P. Accessory Genome Dynamics of Local and Global *Staphylococcus pseudintermedius* Populations. *Front. Microbiol.* **2022**, *13*, 798175. [CrossRef]
27. Viegas, F.M.; Santana, J.A.; Silva, B.A.; Xavier, R.G.C.; Bonisson, C.T.; Câmara, J.L.S.; Rennó, M.C.; Cunha, J.L.R.; Figueiredo, H.C.P.; Lobato, F.C.F.; et al. Occurrence and characterization of methicillin-resistant *Staphylococcus* spp. in diseased dogs in Brazil. *PLoS ONE* **2022**, *17*, e0269422. [CrossRef]
28. Ferrer, L.; García-Fonticoba, R.; Pérez, D.; Viñes, J.; Fàbregas, N.; Madroñero, S.; Meroni, G.; Martino, P.A.; Martínez, S.; Maté, M.L.; et al. Whole genome sequencing and de novo assembly of *Staphylococcus pseudintermedius*: A pangenome approach to unravelling pathogenesis of canine pyoderma. *Vet. Dermatol.* **2021**, *32*, 654–663. [CrossRef]
29. Wegener, A.; Broens, E.M.; van der Graaf-van Bloois, L.; Zomer, A.L.; Visser, C.E.; van Zeijl, J.; van der Meer, C.; Kusters, J.G.; Friedrich, A.W.; Kampinga, G.A.; et al. Absence of Host-Specific Genes in Canine and Human *Staphylococcus pseudintermedius* as Inferred from Comparative Genomics. *Antibiotics* **2021**, *10*, 854. [CrossRef]
30. Sullivan, M.J.; Petty, N.K.; Beatson, S.A. Easyfig: A genome comparison visualizer. *Bioinformatics* **2011**, *27*, 1009–1010. [CrossRef]
31. Bruce, S.A.; Smith, J.T.; Mydosh, J.L.; Ball, J.; Needle, D.B.; Gibson, R.; Andam, C.P. Shared antibiotic resistance and virulence genes in *Staphylococcus aureus* from diverse animal hosts. *Sci. Rep.* **2022**, *12*, 4413. [CrossRef]
32. Worthing, K.A.; Abraham, S.; Coombs, G.W.; Pang, S.; Saputra, S.; Jordan, D.; Trott, D.J.; Norris, J.M. Clonal diversity and geographic distribution of methicillin-resistant *Staphylococcus pseudintermedius* from Australian animals: Discovery of novel sequence types. *Vet. Microbiol.* **2018**, *213*, 58–65. [CrossRef] [PubMed]
33. Pires Dos Santos, T.; Damborg, P.; Moodley, A.; Guardabassi, L. Systematic Review on Global Epidemiology of Methicillin-Resistant *Staphylococcus pseudintermedius*: Inference of Population Structure from Multilocus Sequence Typing Data. *Front. Microbiol.* **2016**, *7*, 1599. [CrossRef] [PubMed]
34. Bannoehr, J.; Ben Zakour, N.L.; Waller, A.S.; Guardabassi, L.; Thoday, K.L.; van den Broek, A.H.; Fitzgerald, J.R. Population genetic structure of the *Staphylococcus intermedius* group: Insights into agr diversification and the emergence of methicillin-resistant strains. *J. Bacteriol.* **2007**, *189*, 8685–8692. [CrossRef]
35. Røken, M.; Iakhno, S.; Haaland, A.H.; Wasteson, Y.; Bjelland, A.M. Transmission of Methicillin-Resistant *Staphylococcus* spp. from Infected Dogs to the Home Environment and Owners. *Antibiotics* **2022**, *11*, 637. [CrossRef]
36. Han, J.I.; Yang, C.H.; Park, H.M. Prevalence and risk factors of *Staphylococcus* spp. carriage among dogs and their owners: A cross-sectional study. *Vet. J.* **2016**, *212*, 15–21. [CrossRef] [PubMed]
37. van Duijkeren, E.; Kamphuis, M.; van der Mije, I.C.; Laarhoven, L.M.; Duim, B.; Wagenaar, J.A.; Houwers, D.J. Transmission of methicillin-resistant *Staphylococcus pseudintermedius* between infected dogs and cats and contact pets, humans and the environment in households and veterinary clinics. *Vet. Microbiol.* **2011**, *150*, 338–343. [CrossRef]
38. Paul, N.C.; Bärgman, S.C.; Moodley, A.; Nielsen, S.S.; Guardabassi, L. *Staphylococcus pseudintermedius* colonization patterns and strain diversity in healthy dogs: A cross-sectional and longitudinal study. *Vet. Microbiol.* **2012**, *160*, 420–427. [CrossRef]
39. Lord, J.; Millis, N.; Jones, R.D.; Johnson, B.; Kania, S.A.; Odoi, A. Patterns of antimicrobial, multidrug and methicillin resistance among *Staphylococcus* spp. isolated from canine specimens submitted to a diagnostic laboratory in Tennessee, USA: A descriptive study. *BMC Vet. Res.* **2022**, *18*, 91. [CrossRef] [PubMed]
40. Moodley, A.; Damborg, P.; Nielsen, S.S. Antimicrobial resistance in methicillin susceptible and methicillin resistant *Staphylococcus pseudintermedius* of canine origin: Literature review from 1980 to 2013. *Vet Microbiol* **2014**, *171*, 337–341. [CrossRef]
41. Abdullahi, I.N.; Zarazaga, M.; Campaña-Burguet, A.; Eguizábal, P.; Lozano, C.; Torres, C. Nasal *Staphylococcus aureus* and *S. pseudintermedius* carriage in healthy dogs and cats: A systematic review of their antibiotic resistance, virulence and genetic lineages of zoonotic relevance. *J. Appl. Microbiol.* **2022**, *133*, 3368–3390. [CrossRef]
42. Mlynarczyk-Bonikowska, B.; Kowalewski, C.; Krolak-Ulinska, A.; Marusza, W. Molecular Mechanisms of Drug Resistance in *Staphylococcus aureus*. *Int. J. Mol. Sci.* **2022**, *23*, 8088. [CrossRef] [PubMed]
43. Bergot, M.; Martins-Simoes, P.; Kilian, H.; Châtre, P.; Worthing, K.A.; Norris, J.M.; Madec, J.-Y.; Laurent, F.; Haenni, M. Evolution of the Population Structure of *Staphylococcus pseudintermedius* in France. *Front. Microbiol.* **2018**, *9*, 3055. [CrossRef] [PubMed]
44. Phumthanakorn, N.; Schwendener, S.; Donà, V.; Chanchaithong, P.; Perreten, V.; Prapasarakul, N. Genomic insights into methicillin-resistant *Staphylococcus pseudintermedius* isolates from dogs and humans of the same sequence types reveals diversity in prophages and pathogenicity islands. *PLoS ONE* **2021**, *16*, e0254382. [CrossRef]
45. Suepaul, S.; Georges, K.; Unakal, C.; Boyen, F.; Sookhoo, J.; Ashraph, K.; Yusuf, A.; Butaye, P. Determination of the frequency, species distribution and antimicrobial resistance of staphylococci isolated from dogs and their owners in Trinidad. *PLoS ONE* **2021**, *16*, e0254048. [CrossRef] [PubMed]
46. Larsen, J.; Enright, M.C.; Godoy, D.; Spratt, B.G.; Larsen, A.R.; Skov, R.L. Multilocus sequence typing scheme for *Staphylococcus aureus*: Revision of the gmk locus. *J. Clin. Microbiol.* **2012**, *50*, 2538–2539. [CrossRef]
47. Kaas, R.S.; Leekitcharoenphon, P.; Aarestrup, F.M.; Lund, O. Solving the problem of comparing whole bacterial genomes across different sequencing platforms. *PLoS ONE* **2014**, *9*, e104984. [CrossRef]
48. Letunic, I.; Bork, P. Interactive Tree Of Life (iTOL) v5: An online tool for phylogenetic tree display and annotation. *Nucleic Acids Res.* **2021**, *49*, W293–W296. [CrossRef]
49. Hasman, H.; Saputra, D.; Sicheritz-Ponten, T.; Lund, O.; Svendsen, C.A.; Frimodt-Møller, N.; Aarestrup, F.M. Rapid whole-genome sequencing for detection and characterization of microorganisms directly from clinical samples. *J. Clin. Microbiol.* **2014**, *52*, 139–146. [CrossRef]

50. Bortolaia, V.; Kaas, R.S.; Ruppe, E.; Roberts, M.C.; Schwarz, S.; Cattoir, V.; Philippon, A.; Allesoe, R.L.; Rebelo, A.R.; Florensa, A.F.; et al. ResFinder 4.0 for predictions of phenotypes from genotypes. *J. Antimicrob. Chemother.* **2020**, *75*, 3491–3500. [CrossRef]
51. Carattoli, A.; Zankari, E.; García-Fernández, A.; Voldby Larsen, M.; Lund, O.; Villa, L.; Møller Aarestrup, F.; Hasman, H. In silico detection and typing of plasmids using PlasmidFinder and plasmid multilocus sequence typing. *Antimicrob. Agents Chemother.* **2014**, *58*, 3895–3903. [CrossRef] [PubMed]
52. Arndt, D.; Grant, J.R.; Marcu, A.; Sajed, T.; Pon, A.; Liang, Y.; Wishart, D.S. PHASTER: A better, faster version of the PHAST phage search tool. *Nucleic Acids Res.* **2016**, *44*, W16–W21. [CrossRef] [PubMed]
53. Chen, L.; Zheng, D.; Liu, B.; Yang, J.; Jin, Q. VFDB 2016: Hierarchical and refined dataset for big data analysis—10 years on. *Nucleic Acids Res.* **2016**, *44*, D694–D697. [CrossRef] [PubMed]

antibiotics

MDPI

Article

Methicillin-Resistant *Staphylococcus aureus* Strains Isolated from Burned Patients in a Tunisian Hospital: Molecular Typing, Virulence Genes, and Antimicrobial Resistance

Souhir Kmiha [1], Ahlem Jouini [1,*], Nahawend Zerriaa [1], Safa Hamrouni [1], Lamia Thabet [2] and Abderrazak Maaroufi [1]

1 Laboratory of Epidemiology and Veterinary Microbiology, Group of Bacteriology and Biotechnology Development, Pasteur Institute of Tunis, University of Tunis El Manar, Tunis 2092, Tunisia; souhirkmiha@yahoo.fr (S.K.)

2 Laboratory of Microbiology, Center for Traumatology and Major Burns, Rue du 1er Mai, Ben Arous 2013, Tunisia; thabetlamia@gmail.com

* Correspondence: ahlem.jouini@pasteur.tn; Tel.: +216-71-783-022

Abstract: Methicillin-resistant *Staphylococcus aureus* (MRSA) is one of the major causes of a variety of infections in hospitals and the community. Their spread poses a serious public health problem worldwide. Nevertheless, in Tunisia and other African countries, very little molecular typing data on MRSA strains is currently available. In our study, a total of 64 MRSA isolates were isolated from clinical samples collected from burned patients hospitalized in the Traumatology and Burns Center of Ben Arous in Tunisia. The identification of the collection was based on conventional methods (phenotypic and molecular characterization). The characterization of the genetic support for methicillin resistance was performed by amplification of the *mecA* gene by polymerase chain reaction (PCR), which revealed that 78.12% of *S. aureus* harbors the gene. The resistance of all the collection to different antibiotic families was studied. Indeed, the analysis of strain antibiotic susceptibility confirmed their multi-resistant phenotype, with high resistance to ciprofloxacin, gentamicin, penicillin, erythromycin, and tetracycline. The resistance to the last three antibiotics was conferred by the *blaZ* gene (73.43%), the *erm*(C) gene (1.56%), the *msr*(*A*) gene (6.25%), and *tet*(*M*) gene (7.81%), respectively. The clonal diversity of these strains was studied by molecular typing of the accessory gene regulator (*agr*) system, characterization of the SCC*mec* type, and *spa*-typing. The results revealed the prevalence of *agr* types II and III groups, the SCC*mec* type III and II cassettes, and the dominance of *spa* type t233. The characterization of the eight enterotoxins genes, the Panton-Valentine leukocidin and the toxic shock syndrome toxin, was determined by PCR. The percentage of virulence genes detected was for enterotoxins (55%), *tst* (71.88%), leukocidin E/D (79.69%), and *pvl* (1.56%) factors. Furthermore, our results revealed that the majority of the strains harbor IEC complex genes (94%) with different types. Our findings highlighted the emergence of MRSA strains with a wide variety of toxins, leukocidin associated with resistance genes, and specific genetic determinants, which could constitute a risk of their spread in hospitals and the environment and complicate infection treatment.

Keywords: Methicillin-resistant *S. aureus* (MRSA); *mecA* gene; virulence factors; *spa* typing; *agr* typing; Panton-Valentine leukocidin; enterotoxins; Tunisia

1. Introduction

The high frequency of *Staphylococcus aureus* infections in burn units constitutes a serious problem for infection treatment. Loss of the functional skin barrier and the depression of the immune responses caused by burns have increased the incidence of various infections [1]. The skin is the first barrier of defense against microbial infection, and it becomes more sensitive once it gets burned. Many pathogens are responsible for burn wound infections, including *Staphylococcus*, *Enterococcus*, *Pseudomonas*, *Acinetobacter*, and fungi [1]. *Staphylococcus aureus* bacteria can cause a wide variety of infections, from minor skin infections to life-threatening infections such as pneumonia, endocarditis, and sepsis. During the last five decades, the overuse of antimicrobial agents in human medicine to treat bacterial infections has favored the emergence of multidrug-resistant bacteria, including MRSA, that have spread as human hospital-acquired pathogens (HA-MRSA) throughout the world [2].

The emergence and transmission of methicillin-resistant *S. aureus* (MRSA) in burn centers results in adverse effects such as prolonged hospitalization, bacteremia or sepsis, and even death, which require further prevention and treatment efforts. In Tunisia, the Traumatology and Burn Center (CTGB) is the only burn center that treats different types of burn wounds.

Methicillin resistance in staphylococci is primary mediated by the expression of the *mecA* gene, or its homologue *mecC*, that contains a diverse type of staphylococcal cassette chromosome *mec* (SCC*mec*), based on a mobile genetic element, and encodes an altered penicillin-binding protein with a very low affinity to β-lactam antibiotics [2]. This emergence of multidrug-resistant strains presents a global health issue. In fact, the World Health Organization predicts that by 2050, bacterial resistance will be responsible for 10 million more deaths than cancer [3].

To date, there is no staphylococcal vaccine, and the alternative antibiotic used as an anti-MRSA is vancomycin. The main objective for successful clinical treatment of bacterial infections depends on the analysis of the antibiotic susceptibility profiles and the antibiotic resistance mechanisms of pathogenic bacteria. In addition to antibiotic resistance, *S. aureus* isolates can harbor a diversity of virulence factor genes, including the Panton-Valentine leukocidin (PVL), the toxic shock syndrome toxin 1 (TSST), and the staphylococcal enterotoxins (SE) [4], immune evasion factors like staphylokinase (Sak), staphylococcal inhibitor of complement (SCIN), and chemotaxis inhibitory protein (CIP), including CHIPS. These virulence factors may contribute to human or animal skin and soft tissue infections, as well as cases of severe pneumonia and food poisoning [4]. The number and combinations of toxin genes may contribute to the pathogenicity of *S. aureus*. It is important to highlight that the expression of virulence genes is under the control of a global quorum-sensing regulator system named *agr* (accessory gene regulator), which is associated with the pathogenesis and molecular typing of antibiotic resistance in *S. aureus* [5]. Mobile genetic elements (MGEs) carrying resistance genes such as plasmids, transposons, and genomic islands frequently harbor virulence factor genes [2,6].

The molecular characterization of *S. aureus* is very interesting for the identification and knowledge of the circulation of virulent and resistant clones in hospital settings [6]. In fact, the most useful typing tool for epidemiological studies of *S. aureus* that gives an excellent discriminatory result is *spa*-typing based on the sequence variation in a hypervariable region of the staphylococcal protein A *spa* gene. The *spa* gene encodes a surface protein that plays a role in the adhesion and colonization of *S. aureus* [7]. The prevalence of *spa* types of *S. aureus* isolates varies among different origins and countries [6,7].

To develop effective control and treatment of human infections, it is important to study the genetic diversity, antimicrobial resistance, and virulence of *S. aureus* associated with infectious diseases. These types of data are limited in Tunisia. Therefore, the aim of this study was to determine the genetic lineages, antibiotic resistance genes, and virulence determinants of *S. aureus* isolates from clinical samples of burned patients in Tunisia.

2. Results

2.1. Confirmation of *S. aureus* Isolates

The biochemical and molecular identification was performed on the sixty-four isolates collected from the Microbiology laboratory of CTGB. All the isolates were identified as *S. aureus* since they presented the ability to coagulate rabbit plasma and were confirmed by a species-specific *nuc* gene PCR assay.

2.2. Antibiotic Resistance Rates

The occurrence of antibiotic resistance in the 64 *S. aureus* isolates is presented in Figure 1. All *S. aureus* strains were confirmed to be MRSA and presented oxacillin and/or cefoxitin resistance. A high resistance rate for the β-lactam, quinolone, and aminoglycoside families was observed. The percentages were as follows: cefoxitin (100%), ciprofloxacin (86%), gentamicin (83%), and penicillin (75%), while moderate and low resistance rates were detected for: fosfomycin (28%), oxacillin (26%), fusidic acid (25%), amikacin (23%), tobramycin (22%), ampicillin (22%), kanamycin (20%), tetracycline (17%), erythromycin (8%), and teicoplanin (1.5%). Sixty *S. aureus* isolates were multiresistant to at least three antibiotic families.

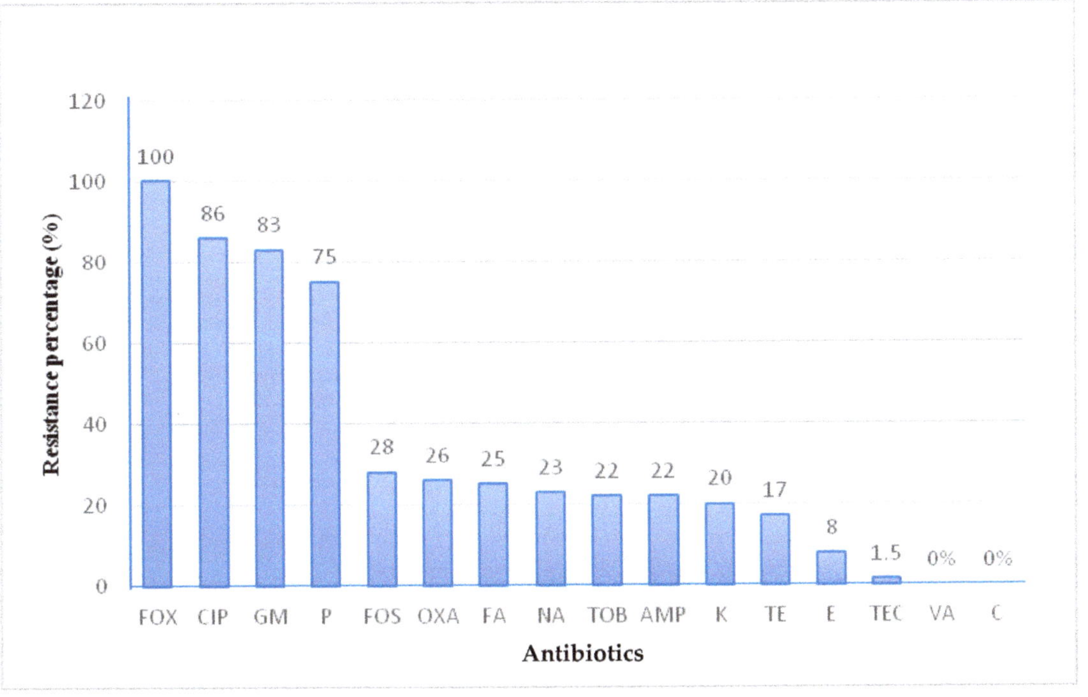

Figure 1. Phenotypic resistance rate of MRSA isolates. Penicillin (P), Oxacillin (OXA), Cefoxitin (FOX), Gentamicin (GM), Kanamycin (K), Tobramycin (TOB), Tetracycline (TE), Ciprofloxacin (CIP), Erythromycin (E), Fusidic Acid (FA), Ampicillin (AMP), Teicoplanin (TEC), Amikacin (NA), Fosfomycin (FOS), Vancomycin (VA) and Chloramphenicol (C).

2.3. Genetic Support of Antibiotic Resistance

The characteristics of resistance genes in *S. aureus* isolates are shown in Figure 2. The molecular characterization of methicillin resistance by PCR amplification showed that 50 MRSA strains harbored the *mecA* gene. Penicillin resistance is coded by the *blaZ* gene in 47 MRSA isolates. Furthermore, tetracycline resistance was conferred by *tet*(*M*) genes in only five isolates; *tet*(*L*) and *tet*(*K*) genes were not detected. For the five erythromycin-resistant MRSA isolates, *erm*(C) gene was detected in only one strain and *msr*(*A*) gene in four isolates. The *erm*(*A*), *erm*(B), and *msr*(*B*) genes were not detected in all the collection.

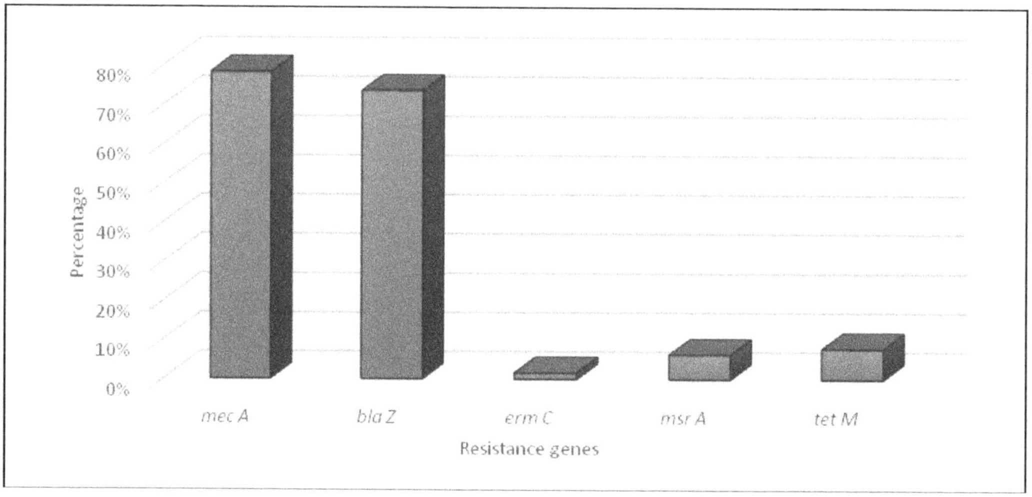

Figure 2. Distribution of antibiotic resistance genes in MRSA isolates.

2.4. Molecular Typing of MRSA Isolates

Table 1 presents molecular typing by SCC*mec* cassettes, *spa*-typing, and *agr*-typing. The characterization of SCC*mec* cassettes was performed by multiplex PCR amplification of genes encoding *ccr* recombination.

The results revealed that 37 of the tested strains (57%) exhibited different *ccr* profiles. Indeed, the most dominant recombination was *ccrA3-ccrB*, assigned to SCC*mec* type III in 22 strains, of which 4 were *mecA* gene negative, followed by *ccrA2-ccrB* recombination assigned to SCC*mec* type II in 13 strains, of which only 1 was *mecA* gene negative. In addition, the *ccrA1-ccrB* recombination allocated to SCC*mec* type I was detected in two MRSA strains, one of which was *mecA*-negative (Table 1).

The analysis of the results of *spa* type for all MRSA strains showed the presence of 10 different *spa* types (*spa* type number of isolates): t233 (20), t2524 (6), t067 (3), t1192 (3), t1209 (3), t037 (3), t2453 (1), t2612 (5), t9082 (1), and t808 (1). Nevertheless, the *spa* type in eighteen strains was not typable.

The amplification of the *agr* locus by multiplex PCR showed the dominance of the *agr* II type in 28 strains, followed by the *agr* III type in 23 strains; the remaining isolates were ascribed to the *agr* I type.

2.5. Virulence Genes and IEC Profile of MRSA Isolates

The presence of virulence genes in MRSA isolates is shown in Table 2 and Figure 3.

Table 1. Molecular typing of MRSA isolates by *ccr* genes, *spa* type, and *agr* type.

Reference of Strains	Origin	System *agr*	*ccr*	*spa* Type	SCC*mec*	*mec* Complex
D354	SV	III	*ccrA2-ccrB*	t233	II	A
H2071/2073	Bc	II	–	NT	–	–
D544	PC	III	–	t067	–	–
D905	PC	III	*ccrA3-ccrB*	t1209	III	A
D1069	PC	III	*ccrA3-ccrB*	NT	III	A
D2435	PB	III	*ccrA1-ccrB*	t067	I	B
D21	PB	III	*ccrA2-ccrB*	NT	II	A

Table 1. *Cont.*

Reference of Strains	Origin	System *agr*	*ccr*	*spa* Type	SCC*mec*	*mec* Complex
H1240	Bc	II	*ccrA3-ccrB*	NT	III	A
D210	PB	I	*ccrA3-ccrB*	t2453	III	A
D1462	PB	II	*ccrA2-ccrB*	t9082	II	A
H1066	Bc	III	–	NT	–	–
D1719	PC	III	*ccrA2-ccrB*	t233	II	A
D1434	PC	III	–	t1209	–	–
D1065	PC	II	*ccrA3-ccrB*	t067	III	A
D976	PC	I	–	t2524	–	–
D847	PC	II	*ccrA2-ccrB*	NT	II	A
D2367	PC	II	–	t233	–	–
1039	PC	II	*ccrA2-ccrB*	t1209	II	A
H3720/3772	Bc	II	*ccrA2-ccrB*	t233	II	A
D2085	PC	II	*ccrA3-ccrB*	t233	III	A
H930	Bc	I	*ccrA2-ccrB*	NT	II	A
D1467	PC	II		t2612	–	–
D2376	PC	II	*ccrA2-ccrB*	NT	II	A
H405	Bc	I	–	NT	–	–
H745	Bc	I	*ccrA3-ccrB*	NT	III	A
D2377	PC	II	*ccrA2-ccrB*	t037	II	A
H3715	Bc	III	*ccrA3-ccrB*	t2612	III	A
D2504	KTY	III	*ccrA3-ccrB*	t2612	III	A
D1060	PC	III	*ccrA3-ccrB*	NT	III	A
H950	Bc	III	*ccrA2-ccrB*	t233	II	A
D1114	PC	II	–	t233	–	–
D1829	SV	III	*ccrA3-ccrB*	t233	III	A
D60	KTY	III	–	t233	–	–
D942	CBES	I	–	t233	–	–
D675	PC	III	–	t233	–	–
D1880	PC	II	–	t233	–	–
D1388	PC	III	–	t233	–	–
H794	Bc	II	–	t037	–	–
D1095	NP	II	–	t233	–	–
D1124	PC	III	–	t2524	–	–
H73	Bc	II	–	t233	–	–
H3741	Bc	II	*ccrA3-ccrB*	t2612	III	A
D2240	PC	II		t2612	–	–
D2252	PC	II	*ccrA2-ccrB*	t2524	II	A
H814	Bc	III	*ccrA1-ccrB*	NT	I	B
D1691	PC	I	–	t233	–	–
D1363	KTY	III	*ccrA3-ccrB*	t808	III	A

Table 1. *Cont.*

Reference of Strains	Origin	System *agr*	*ccr*	*spa* Type	SCC*mec*	*mec* Complex
D491	CBES	I	*ccrA3-ccrB*	NT	III	A
H2268	PC	I	–	t037	–	–
H2879	Bc	II	*ccrA3-ccrB*	NT	III	A
D2187	PC	III	*ccrA3-ccrB*	t2524	III	A
D48	KTY	III	*ccrA3-ccrB*	t233	III	A
D1128	PC	I	*ccrA3-ccrB*	NT	III	A
D1971	KTY	I	*ccrA3-ccrB*	NT	III	A
D890	KTY	I	–	NT	–	–
D1747	PC	II	–	t1192	–	–
H3008	Bc	II	*ccrA3-ccrB*	t1192	III	A
D1077	PC	II	–	t2524	–	–
H1042	Bc	III	*ccrA2-ccrB*	t1192	II	A
D2393	PC	I	–	t2524	–	–
H793	Bc	II	*ccrA3-ccrB*	t233	III	A
H782	Bc	II	–	NT	–	–
D1033	CBES	II	–	t233	–	–
D1836/1795	PC	II	–	t233	–	–

Bc: Blood culture; PC: Post cibum; PB: Puncture; CBES: Cytobacteriological examination of sputum; NP: Nasal pus; KTY, KTV: Catheter; SV: Septum. NT: not typable; SCC*mec*: Staphylococcal Cassette Chromosome *mec*; *Spa*: *S. aureus* protein A; *agr*: accessory gene regulator; *ccr*: cassette chromosome recombinase.

Table 2. Resistance phenotype profiles, resistance genes, *agr*-typing, virulence factors, and the Immune Evasion Cluster detected in MRSA isolates.

Reference of Strains	Origin	Antibiotic-Resistant Phenotype	Resistance Genes Detected	Virulence Factors	*agr* System
D354	SV	OXA, CIP, GM, FOX, FA	*mecA-blaZ*	*tst, seg, sea, see*, IEC B	III
H2071/2073	Bc	OXA, CIP, GM, FOX, FA	*mecA-blaZ*	IEC E, *seo, tst*	II
D544	PC	FOX, OXA	*mecA*	leucocidin E/D, IEC B, *sem, sea, see, tst*	III
D905	PC	OXA, CIP, GM, FOX	*mecA-blaZ*	*sei, sea, see, seo, tst*, IEC B	III
D1069	PC	OXA, FA, CIP, GM, FOX	*blaZ*	*tst*, IEC B	III
D2435	PB	OXA, FOX	*blaZ*	*tst*	III
D21	PB	OXA, FOX, FA	*mecA*	leucocidin E/D, Panton Valentine leucocidin, *tst*, IEC D	III
H1240	Bc	OXA, FA, GM, FOX	*mecA-blaZ*	*tst*, IEC E	II
D210	PB	OXA, FA	*mecA*	*tst*, IEC E	I
D1462	PB	OXA, P, CIP, GM, TOB, K, FOX, NA, AMP, TE, E	*mecA-blaZ-erm(C)*	leucocidin E/D, Panton Valentine leucocidin, *tst, sem, sea, see*, IEC B	II

Table 2. *Cont.*

Reference of Strains	Origin	Antibiotic-Resistant Phenotype	Resistance Genes Detected	Virulence Factors	*agr* System
H1066	Bc	OXA, FA, CIP, FOX	*mecA-blaZ*	leucocidin E/D, *tst*, IEC D	III
D1719	PC	CIP, GM, FOX	*mecA-blaZ*	leucocidin E/D, *tst*, IEC (*scn*, *sak*, *sea*, *sep*)	III
D1434	PC	OXA, CIP, GM, FOX	*blaZ*	leucocidin E/D, *tst*, IEC B	III
D1065	PC	OXA, FOX	*mecA-blaZ*	leucocidin E/D, *tst*, IEC (*sak*, *chp*)	II
D976	PC	FA, CIP, GM, FOX	*mecA-blaZ*	leucocidin PV, *tst*, IEC E	I
D847	PC	OXA, P, CIP, GM, TOB, K, FOX, NA, AMP, TE	*mecA-blaZ*	leucocidin E/D, *tst*, *sem*, *sea*, *see*, IEC B	II
D2367	PC	CIP, GM, FOX	*mecA*	leucocidin E/D, *tst*, *sem*, *sea*, *see*, IEC B	II
1039	PC	OXA, CIP, GM, FOX	*mecA-blaZ*	leucocidin E/D, *tst*, *sem*, *sea*, *see*, IEC B	II
H3720/3772	Bc	CIP, GM, FOX	*mecA-blaZ*	leucocidin E/D, IEC E	II
D2085	PC	CIP, GM, FOX	*mecA-blaZ*	leucocidin E/D, *tst*, *sem*, *sea*, *see*, IEC B	II
H930	Bc	GM, FOX, TEC	*mecA-blaZ*	leucocidin E/D, *tst*, IEC E	I
D1467	PC	FOX, CIP, GM, FOX	*mecA-blaZ*	leucocidin E/D, *tst*, IEC B	II
D2376	PC	FOX, NA, AMP, P	*blaZ*	leucocidin E/D, *tst*, *sei*, *seo*, *sea*, *see*, IEC B	II
H405	Bc	FOS, FA, CIP, FOX	*mecA-blaZ*	leucocidin E/D, *tst*, IEC B	I
H745	Bc	FOS, FA, CIP, FOX, GM	*mecA-blaZ*	leucocidin E/D, *tst*, *sen*, *sea*, *see*, IEC (*chp*)	I
D2377	PC	FOS, CIP, FOX	*mecA-blaZ*	leucocidin E/D, *tst*, *seo*, *sea*, *see*, IEC B	II
H3715	Bc	FOS, FA, CIP, FOX, GM	*mecA-blaZ*	leucocidin E/D, *tst*, *seg*, *sem*, *see*, *sea*, IEC B	III
D2504	KTY	FOS, FA, CIP, FOX, GM	*mecA-blaZ*	leucocidin E/D, *tst*, *seg*, *sem*, *see*, *sea*, IEC B	III
D1060	PC	CIP, GM, TOB, K, FOX, NA,	*mecA-blaZ*	leucocidin E/D, *tst*, *seg*, *sem*, *see*, *sea*, IEC B	III
H950	Bc	CIP, GM, FOX	*mecA-blaZ*	leucocidin E/D, *tst*, IEC B	III
D1114	PC	CIP, GM, FOX	-	leucocidin E/D, *tst*, *seg*, *sem*, *see*, *sea*, IEC E	II
D1829	SV	CIP, GM, FOX	*mecA*	leucocidin E/D, *seg*, *sem*, *see*, *sea*, *sen*, IEC (*sak*, *chp*)	III
D60	KTY	CIP, GM, FOX	*mecA-blaZ*	leucocidin E/D, *seg*,*sem*, *see*, *sea*, IEC (*sak*, *chp*, *scn*, *sea*)	III

Table 2. *Cont.*

Reference of Strains	Origin	Antibiotic-Resistant Phenotype	Resistance Genes Detected	Virulence Factors	*agr* System
D942	CBES	CIP, GM, FOX	*mecA-blaZ*	leucocidin E/D, *seg*, *seu*, *see*, *sea*, IEC B	I
D675	PC	CIP, GM, FOX	*mecA*	leucocidin E/D, *tst*, *sei*, *seo*, IEC (*sak*, *scn*, *sep*, *sea*)	III
D1880	PC	CIP, GM, FOX	*mecA*	leucocidin E/D, *tst*, *seg*, *sem*, *seu*, *sea*, *see*, IEC (*sak*)	II
D1388	PC	CIP, GM, FOX	*blaZ*	leucocidin E/D, Panton Valentine leucocidin, *tst*, *seo*, *sem*, *seu*, *sea*, *see*, *sei*, IEC B	III
H794	Bc	FOS, CIP, FOX	*mecA*	leucocidin E/D, *sem*, *see*, *sea*, IEC (*sak*, *chp*)	II
D1095	NP	FA, CIP, GM, TOB, K, FOX, NA, AMP, P, TE, E	*mecA-msrA*	leucocidin E/D, *sem*, *see*, *sea*, *seu*, IEC (*sak*, *chp*)	II
D1124	PC	FA, CIP, GM, FOX	*mecA*	leucocidin E/D, *tst*, IEC B	III
H73	Bc	CIP, GM, FOX	*mecA*	leucocidin E/D, IEC (*sea*)	II
H3741	Bc	CIP, GM, FOX, FOS	*mecA*	leucocidin E/D, IEC (*sak*, *chp*, *scn*)	II
D2240	PC	CIP, GM, FOX, FOS	*mecA-blaZ*	leucocidin E/D, IEC (*chp*)	II
D2252	PC	CIP, GM, FOX, FA	*mecA*	leucocidin E/D, IEC (*scn*), *tst*	II
H814	Bc	CIP, GM, FOX, FOS, FA	*mecA-blaZ*	leucocidin E/D, IEC (*scn*), *tst*, *sea*, *see*	III
D1691	PC	CIP, GM, FOX	-	leucocidin E/D, *tst*, IEC B	I
D1363	KTY	FA, CIP, GM, TOB, K, FOX, AMP, P, TE	*mecA-blaZ*	leucocidin E/D, *tst*, *sem*, *see*, *seu*, *sea*, IEC D	III
D491	CBES	CIP, GM, TOB, K, FOX, NA, AMP, TE	*blaZ*	*tst*, *sem*, *see*, *seu*, *sea*, IEC B	I
H2268	PC	CIP, GM, TOB, K, FOX, NA, AMP, TE, FOS, P, E	*mecA-blaZ-tet(M)-msr(A)*	-	I
H2879	Bc	CIP, GM, TOB, FOX, NA, AMP, TE, FOS, P, E	*mecA-blaZ-msrA*	leucocidin E/D, IEC (*sak*), *tst*	II
D2187	PC	CIP, GM, FOX, FOS	*mecA-blaZ*	leucocidin E/D, *tst*	III
D48	KTY	CIP, GM, FOX, NA	*blaZ*	leucocidin E/D, *tst*	III
D1128	PC	CIP, GM, TOB, K, FOX, NA, AMP, P	*mecA-blaZ*	leucocidin E/D, *tst*, IEC B	I
D1971	KTY	CIP, GM, TOB, K, FOX, NA, AMP, P, TE, E	*mecA-blaZ-tet(M)-msrA*	leucocidin E/D, *tst*, IEC B	I
D890	KTY	CIP, GM, TOB, K, FOX, NA, AMP, P	*mecA-blaZ*	*tst*, *seg*, *seu*, *sea*, *see*, IEC B	I

Table 2. *Cont.*

Reference of Strains	Origin	Antibiotic-Resistant Phenotype	Resistance Genes Detected	Virulence Factors	*agr* System
D1747	PC	CIP, GM, TOB, K, FOX, NA, AMP, P, TE	*blaZ-tet(M)*	*sem, seu, sea, see*, IEC B	II
H3008	Bc	CIP, GM, FOX, TOB, K, NA, AMP, P, TE	*mecA-blaZ-tet(M)*	leucocidin E/D, *seg, seu, sea, see*, IEC (*chp*)	II
D1077	PC	GM, FOX, CIP, FOS	*mecA-blaZ*	*tst*, IEC (*sak, chp*)	II
H1042	Bc	CIP, GM, TOB, K, FOX, NA, AMP, P, TE	*mecA-blaZ-tet(M)*	leucocidin E/D, *sem, seu, sea, see*, IEC B	III
D2393	PC	GM, FOX, CIP, FOS	*mecA*	*seg, seu, sea, see*, IEC B	I
H793	Bc	GM, FOX, CIP	*blaZ*	leucocidin E/D, *seg, seu, sea, see*, IEC B	II
H782	Bc	GM, FOX, CIP, FOS, FA	-	leucocidin E/D, *sea, see*, IEC (*chp*)	II
D1033	CBES	GM, FOX, CIP	*blaZ*	leucocidin E/D, *seg, seu, sea, see*, IEC B	II
D1836/1795	PC	GM, FOX, CIP	*blaZ*	leucocidin E/D, *seu, sea, see*, IEC E	II

Bc: Blood culture; PC: Post cibum; PB: Puncture; CBES: Cytobacteriological examination of sputum; NP: Nasal pus; KTY, KTV: Catheter; SV: Septum. Enterotoxin genes (*sem, seu, sea, see, seg*), toxic shock syndrome toxin 1 (*tst*), immune evasion cluster (IEC) system, leukocidin of Panton Valentine (PVL, *lukF-lukS*-PV). *mecA*: gene encoding methicillin resistance; *blaZ*: gene encoding penicillin resistance; *tet(M)*: gene encoding tetracycline resistance; *msr(A)*: gene encoding erythromycin and clindamycin resistance; *erm(C)*: gene encoding erythromycin resistance. Penicillin (P), Oxacillin (OXA), Cefoxitin (FOX), Gentamicin (GM), Kanamycin (K), Tobramycin (TOB), Tetracycline (TE), Ciprofloxacin (CIP), Erythromycin (E), Fusidic Acid (FA), Ampicillin (AMP), Teicoplanin (TEC), Amikacin (AN), Fosfomycin (FOS).

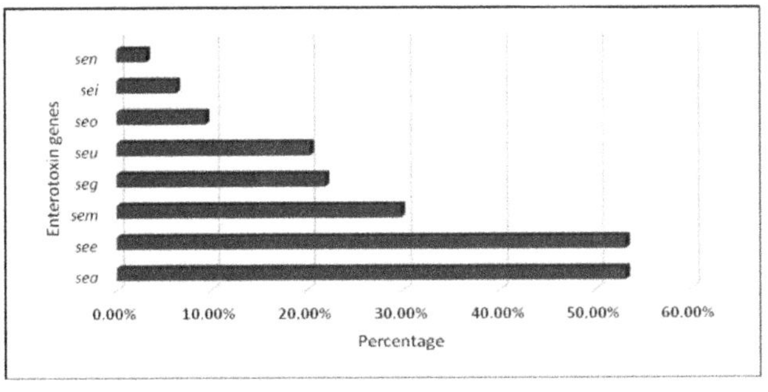

(**a**)

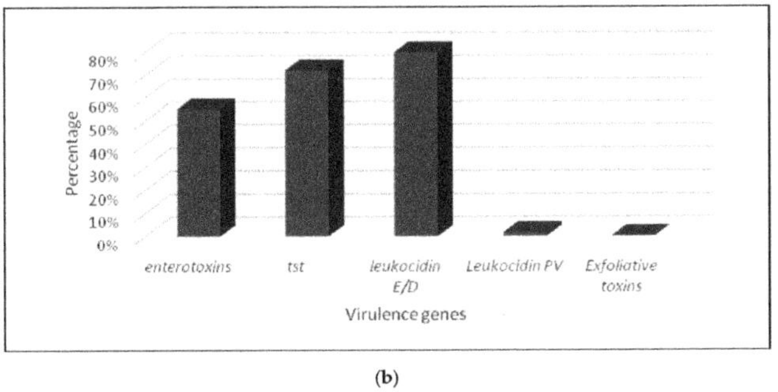

(**b**)

Figure 3. Prevalence of virulence genes in MRSA isolates: (**a**) enterotoxins and (**b**) different virulence genes.

The multiplex PCR of different virulence factors revealed that 63 MRSA isolates (98.44%) harbored virulence genes. Eight enterotoxin genes were detected (number of isolates, percentage) (Figure 3a): *seg* (14, 21.87%), *sea* (34, 53.12%), *see* (34, 53.12%), *seo* (6, 9.37%), *sem* (19, 29.68%), *sei* (4, 6.25%), *sen* (2, 3.12%), and *seu* (13, 20.31%). While the genes coding for the toxic shock protein TSST were found in 46 (71.88%) strains, four MRSA harbored the gene *lukS-lukF* encoding for PVL and were associated with leukocidin E/D factor in three strains. In addition, 51 isolates carried the gene for leukocidin E/D factor; none of them was *etA*- or *etB*-positive (Figure 3b). Different gene combinations coding the IEC complex were found in almost all *S. aureus* strains (n = 60) and assigned to 3 IEC types: IEC type B with the association of *scn*, *sak*, and *chp*; type E with the association of *scn* and *sak*; and type D with the association of *scn*, *sak*, and *sea*.

3. Discussion

Staphylococcus aureus is one of the main causes of nosocomial and hospital infections, leading to serious health problems [2]. Our study focused on the characterization of antibiotic resistance, mainly methicillin resistance, in *S. aureus* strains isolated from different clinical samples of burned patients hosted in the Burn and Traumatology Center in Tunisia. The research on the genetic support of various resistance mechanisms and virulence factors, as well as molecular typing, was intended to provide insight into their clonal diversity and the spread of resistant and virulent clones. Our study included 64 *staphylococcus* strains recovered from clinical samples taken from burned patients. Biochemical and molecular identification revealed that all isolates are *staphylococcus aureus*. The presence of *S. aureus* in burned patients in the Tunisian Center could indicate that this species is involved in cutaneous superinfections of burns due to its commensalism and its diverse virulence factors. Our results are in agreement with those of the study of Thabet et al. [8], performed in two Tunisian hospital structures (CTGB and Aziza Othman Tunis) and reporting that *S. aureus* is the main bacteria isolated in burns in the new hospital center. Its implication in different types of infections was in agreement with recent reports from China, Iran, and Africa describing *S. aureus* as the main pathogen bacteria frequently isolated from burned patients and hospital settings [6].

The analysis of antibiotic resistance in the current study revealed that all strains have been confirmed to be methicillin-resistant. This could be due to the widespread and uncontrolled use of β-lactam drugs, which are the first-line treatment for staphylococcal infection [9]. Our feeding is in agreement with different studies in Tunisia [10–12], Morocco [13], and Africa [6]. This resistance to beta-lactams has evolved in successive waves as specific resistance mechanisms have been acquired [14]. In the same context, Fallagas et al. [15] showed that in most of the high and medium Human Development Index countries analyzed, the most pronounced increase was observed in Tunisia, with an increase up to 41–46% after 2005, as compared with a prevalence of 12%–18% years before. Thus far, in South Africa, the prevalence of MRSA decreased from 36% in 2006 to 24% during 2007–2011, probably due to the implementation of effective infection control policies. In Algeria and Egypt, according to the same study, the prevalence of MRSA between 2003 and 2005 was 45% and 52%, respectively. Morocco is the only country where a low prevalence of MRSA seems to have stabilized during 2003–2008.

The MRSA strains showed high resistance to all β-lactam antibiotics. The molecular analysis of methicillin resistance showed that 78% of MRSA isolates harbored the *mecA* gene; the remaining strains (22%) were *mecA*-negative; this suggests that they may contain further variant cassette genes of the *mecA* gene, such as the *mecC*, *mecB*, or *mecD* genes recently detected [2]. Indeed, the dissemination of MRSA encoded by the *mecA* gene in clinical settings has been reported in various African and European countries. This resistance has emerged through the SCC*mec* cassette genes, which can disseminate by horizontal transfer [16].

In addition to the resistance to methicillin, MRSA isolates showed resistance, especially to penicillin, conferred by the *blaZ* gene (73.43% of isolates). The resistance to tetracycline and erythromycin is encoded, respectively, by *tet(M)*, *erm*(C), and *msr(A)* genes. Our findings conflict with the study of Zmantar et al. [17], which reported a higher frequency of *erm(A)* and *erm*(C) genes detected in MRSA isolates from the oral cavity of Tunisian children. Nevertheless, our results were similar to those of Mkhize et al. [17], who described the presence of the *erm*(C) gene and the absence of the *erm(A)* and *erm(B)* genes in *S. aureus* isolates collected from public hospitals in South Africa [18].

The characterization of SCC*mec* types in our analyzed collection by multiplex PCR amplification of genes encoding *ccr* recombination revealed that 37 strains (57%) exhibited different *ccr* profiles. Indeed, the most dominant recombination was *ccrA3-ccrB*, assigned to SCC*mec* type III (3A), followed by the *ccrA2-ccrB* recombination assigned to SCC*mec* type II (2A), with only two strains having the *ccrA1-ccrB* recombination (SCC*mec* type I (1A)). Nevertheless, SCC*mec* types I, II, and III were the most common during a study conducted at Charles Nicole Hospital in Tunis [19] and SCC*mec* type IV is the most often reported cassette in the majority of research performed in clinical settings in Tunisia [6,10,11,20].

Furthermore, SCC*mec* type I was also reported in the hospital environment in Tunisia [21]. Chen K. et al. [1] demonstrated that the most prevalent clone of MRSA in the burn center in Southeastern China was ST239-SCC*mec*III-t030. According to research performed in Brazil in 2013, SCC*mec* type III had the highest prevalence in burn units [22]. Nevertheless, another study in Iran reported several types of SCC*mec* (47.5% type III, 25% type IV, 10% type V, 10% type II, and 7.5% type I) in MRSA isolates from burned patients at Motahari Hospital (Iran) [23].

In the present study, the molecular characterization of the polymorphic X region of the *spa* gene showed the presence of 10 different *spa* types (t233, t2524, t067, t1192, t1209, t037, t2453, t2612, t9082, and t808) among 46 MRSA isolates. Noteworthy, the *spa* type t233 was the most prevalent in 20 MRSA isolates. These findings are not consistent with those reported in a recent study that described the distribution of the most prevalent *spa* types in the world. Indeed, in Africa, t037, t064, and t084 are frequently found. In Europe, it is rather the t032, t008, and t002, and in Asia, the *spa* type t037 and t002 are the most often reported [24]. This suggests that the *spa* type t233 could be a new clone circulating in the CTGB hospital environment.

The molecular typing by amplification of the *agr* locus revealed the dominance of *agr* types II and III, which is in agreement with the study of Kechrid et al. (2011) at the Children's Hospital of Tunis [11]. On the other hand, the study reported by Elhani et al. [25] as well as that of Gharsa et al. [21] showed that the *agr* I group was the most present. The pathogenic and biofilm growth of *S. aureus* are primarily regulated by the accessory gene regulator (*agr*) quorum-sensing system. In a cell density-dependent manner, this system inhibits the transcription of numerous cell wall-associated proteins, such as protein A and microbial surface components recognizing adhesive matrix molecules (MSCRAMMs), and activates a number of exoproteins, such as hemolysins, exfoliative toxins (ETs), and toxic shock syndrome toxins (TSSTs) [26]. Numerous investigations have documented the association between particular *agr* classes, particular clonal complexes, disease kinds, and associated virulence factors. For instance, Holtfreter et al. [27] discovered a correlation between particular *S. aureus* lineages and different *agr* types. Many studies showed that TSST-1 was predominately carried by *agr* III-type isolates, while phages and plasmids commonly occur in *agr* IV isolates that contain *etA* or *etB* genes [28]. The *agr* I type was also the most typical type, particularly among MRSA isolates [28].

Investigation of the virulence determinants and their implication in the infection by MRSA isolates was scarce in Tunisia and Africa. To the best of our knowledge, the current study was the first to characterize the virulence factors in MRSA strains isolated from hospital patients, especially burned ones. Indeed, our findings highlighted the occurrence of MRSA strains with a wider range of virulence genes. The enterotoxin genes were detected in the majority of strains, indicating that despite the fact that enterotoxin genes are encoded by a bacteriophage, the bacteriophage has spread easily among strains with the same genetic background [29]. In addition, we detected that all strains have a high incidence of *sea* and *see* genes, which was in accord with other findings [30].

According to the characterization of virulence factors in our collection, the prevalence of the *lukF/S-PV* gene was low (1.56%). In the same context, Viquez-Molina et al. [31] detected the *lukF/S-PV* gene in 6.9% of *S. aureus* isolated from patients with diabetic foot infections; however, another study from Lisbon did not detect the *lukF/S-PV* gene from the same origin [32]. Many researchers have suggested that the *PVL* locus is carried on a bacteriophage, and this locus is associated with skin infections and occasionally severe necrotizing pneumonia [33,34]. The presence of *PVL* gene in MRSA strains was mostly associated with skin and soft tissue infections and community-associated clones [6]. Reported data from Tunisia and Algeria described high PVL prevalence in MRSA isolates, while studies from South Africa revealed low prevalence [6].

The toxic shock syndrome (TSST), which is generated by *Staphylococcus aureus*, has been associated with a number of acute illnesses [35]. The *tst* gene was found to have a very high percentage in all strains (71.88%). Our results contradicted other research [36] that described a high prevalence of *tst*-carrying isolates among methicillin-susceptible isolates as compared to MRSA isolates, indicating a possible link between the drug resistance of the strains and the occurrence of their virulence genes. In addition, our results reported that *tsst* toxin is produced by MRSA strains affiliated with *agr* types I, II, and III, whereas other research reported that *tsst* is produced preferentially by isolates harboring *agr* III in MRSA strains isolated from hospitals [28].

The genes encoding *etA* and *etB* exfoliatins were no longer detected in our collection; this can be suggested by the fact that the plasmids and phages carrying these exfoliatins are linked to isolates expressing *agr* type IV [28].

There is evidence that some *agr* types are associated with many clinical characteristics. Most toxic shock syndrome (TSST-1) strains, for instance, are classified as *agr* group III, while most strains with leukocidin-induced necrotizing pneumonia are classified as *agr* group II [37,38]. In our study, *lukE/D* was related to *agr* type III. Our findings disagree with the report of Ben Nejma et al. [10], who have revealed that PVL negative strains are classified as *agr* type III. Similarly, Xu et al. [31] demonstrated that all *lukS/F-PV*-positive isolates belong to *agr* group I.

4. Material and Methods

4.1. Bacterial Isolates

The study was carried out on a collection of 64 non-duplicated *S. aureus* isolates collected from 64 different clinical samples from burned patients hospitalized in the Traumatology and Burn Center (CTGB) of Tunisia between January and December 2016. The clinical samples were distributed as follows: blood culture (18), cytobacteriological examination of sputum (3), puncture (4), nasal pus (1), catheters (6), and sebum (32).

The isolates were recovered on petri dishes of Brain Heart Infusion Agar (BHI) from the Microbiology laboratory of CTGB and transferred to the laboratory in a cooler for analysis.

4.2. Strain Identification

The isolates were identified by conventional biochemical tests (Gram staining oxidase, catalase, DNase, and ability to coagulate rabbit plasma (Bio-Rad, France) [4,39]. Molecular identification was performed by species-specific PCR amplification of the *nuc* gene, as previously described [39], with *S. aureus* (ATCC 43300) being used as a control strain.

4.3. Antimicrobial Susceptibility Testing

The determination of antibiotic susceptibility was performed using the disk diffusion method in accordance with the Clinical and Laboratory Standards Institute (CLSI) recommendations [40]. The antimicrobial agents tested (charge in µg) were as follows: penicillin (10), oxacillin (1), cefoxitin (30), vancomycin (30), gentamicin (10), kanamycin (30), tobramycin (10), tetracycline (30), ciprofloxacin (5), erythromycin (15), amikacin, fusidic acid (10), teicoplanin (30), fosfomycin (200), chloramphenicol (30), and ampicillin (30).

4.4. Detection of the mecA Gene

Methicillin resistance was detected by oxacillin and cefoxitin susceptibilities on disk diffusion agar, according to CLSI [40]. Confirmation of methicillin resistance was performed by conventional PCR targeting the *mecA* gene [41]. *S. aureus* ATCC 43300 was used as a control strain.

4.5. SCCmec-Typing in MRSA Isolates

The presence of SCC*mec* types I to V was investigated in MRSA isolates by PCR of the *ccr* recombinases (1–5) and the *mec* gene complex type (A to C), as recommended by the International Working Group on the Classification of Staphylococcal Cassette Chromosome Elements (IWG-SCC) [42] (Table S1).

4.6. Molecular Typing of S. aureus Isolates

S. aureus protein A *spa*-typing was performed in all *S. aureus* isolates (n = 64) as elsewhere described [43]. The polymorphic X region of the *spa* gene was amplified by PCR, sequenced, and analyzed using Ridom *staph*-type software version 1.5.21 (Ridom GmbH). It automatically detects *spa* repeats and assigns a *spa* type, according to http://spaserver.ridom.de/ (accessed on 10 December 2005). To determine the type of *agr* in MRSA, two multiplex PCRs were performed; the first one allowed the amplification of *agr* types I and II, and the second PCR amplified *agr* types III and IV [44].

4.7. Detection of Antimicrobial Resistance Genes

The detection of antimicrobial resistance genes (*blaZ*, *erm(A)*, *erm(B)*, *erm(C)*, *msr(A)*, *msr(B)*, *tet(K)*, *tet(M)*, *and tet(L)*) was investigated in resistant isolates by specific PCRs [45]. Positive and negative controls used in each PCR assay were from the collection of the laboratory of Institute Pasteur of Tunis.

4.8. Detection of Staphylococcal Toxin Genes

All isolates were tested by PCR for the presence of genes coding for the various staphylococcal enterotoxins (*sea*, *see*, *seg*, *sei*, *sem*, *sen*, *seo*, and *seu*), toxic shock syndrome toxin 1 (*tst*), leukocidin of Panton Valentine (PVL, *lukF-lukS-PV*), and exfoliative ETA and ETB toxins (*etA* and *etB*) [46].

4.9. Detection of the Immune Evasion Gene Cluster

All isolates were tested by PCR for the presence of five genes (*scn*, *chp*, *sak*, *sea*, and *sep*) of the immune evasion cluster (IEC) system. These genes are enclosed in the φ3 bacteriophage and encode the IEC system, which helps bacteria survive in the human host by evading the innate immune system. Detected alleles allowed the classification of seven IEC types (from A to G) [47], Table S2.

5. Conclusions

In this study, all the isolates from clinical samples of burned patients were confirmed as MRSA with high rates of resistance to ciprofloxacin and gentamicin conferred by different antibiotic resistance genes. In addition, our data reported the detection of resistance genes and a different virulence profile in MRSA isolates. It is important to report the molecular diversity of *spa* and *agr* types in the study collection.

This genetic diversity can lead to the emergence and spread of virulent and drug resistant clones within the hospital. Therefore, enhanced antimicrobial surveillance efforts are needed to control and regulate the use of antimicrobials in Tunisian hospital settings in order to reduce the risks associated with the acquisition of multidrug-resistant clones containing virulence determinants and the spread of pathogenic bacteria in humans and their environment.

Supplementary Materials: The following supporting information can be downloaded at: https://www.mdpi.com/article/10.3390/antibiotics12061030/s1. Table S1: Different SCCmec types identified in S. aureus. Table S2: IEC type detected according to the combination of five genes (*scn*, *chp*, *sak*, *sea*, and *sep*) of the immune evasion cluster (IEC) system in *S. aureus*.

Author Contributions: Conceptualization, A.J.; methodology, S.K., A.J., N.Z., S.H. and L.T.; validation, A.J.; formal analysis, A.J. and N.Z.; investigation, A.J., S.K. and N.Z.; resources, S.H. and A.M.; writing–original draft, S.K.; writing–review and editing, S.K., A.J. and A.M.; supervision, A.J. and A.M.; project administration, A.J. and A.M.; funding acquisition, A.M. All authors have read and agreed to the published version of the manuscript.

Funding: This work was supported by the Tunisian Ministry of Higher Education, Scientific Research, and Technology (LR16IPT03).

Institutional Review Board Statement: Not applicable.

Informed Consent Statement: Not applicable.

Data Availability Statement: Not applicable.

Acknowledgments: The authors acknowledge Abdeljelil Ghram for his effort in English editing.

Conflicts of Interest: The authors declare no conflict of interest.

References

1. Chen, K.; Lin, S.; Li, P.; Song, Q.; Luo, D.; Liu, T.; Zeng, L.; Zhang, W. Characterization of *Staphylococcus aureus* Isolated from Patients with Burns in a Regional Burn Center, Southeastern China. *BMC. Infect. Dis.* **2018**, *18*, 51. [CrossRef]
2. Lakhundi, S.; Zhang, K. Methicillin-Resistant *Staphylococcus aureus*: Molecular Characterization, Evolution, and Epidemiology. *Clin. Microbiol. Rev.* **2018**, *31*, e00020-18. [CrossRef] [PubMed]
3. World Health Organization. New Report Calls for Urgent Action to Avert Antimicrobial Resistance Crisis. Available online: https://www.who.int/news/item/29-04-2019 (accessed on 29 April 2020).
4. Fisher, E.L.; Otto, M.; Cheung, G.Y.C. Basis of Virulence in Enterotoxin-Mediated Staphylococcal Food Poisoning. *Front. Microbiol.* **2018**, *9*, 436. [CrossRef]
5. Jenul, C.; Horswill, A.R. Regulation of *Staphylococcus aureus* Virulence. *Microbiol. Spectr.* **2019**, *7*, 2. [CrossRef] [PubMed]
6. Abdulgader, S.M.; Shittu, A.O.; Nicol, M.P.; Kaba, M. Molecular Epidemiology of Methicillin-Resistant *Staphylococcus aureus* in Africa: A Systematic Review. *Front. Microbiol.* **2015**, *6*, 348. [CrossRef] [PubMed]
7. O'Hara, F.P.; Suaya, J.A.; Ray, G.T.; Baxter, R.; Brown, M.L.; Mera, R.M.; Close, N.M.; Thomas, E.; Amrine-Madsen, H. *Spa* typing and multilocus sequence typing show comparable performance in a macroepidemiologic study of *Staphylococcus aureus* in the United States. *Microb. Drug Resist.* **2016**, *22*, 88–96. [CrossRef] [PubMed]
8. Thabet, L.; Zoghlami, A.; Boukadida, J.; Ghanem, A.; Messadi, A.A. Comparative study of antibiotic resistance in bacteria isolated from burned patients during two periods (2005–2008, 2008–2011) and in two hospitals (Hospital Aziza Othmana, Trauma and Burn Center). *Tunis. Med.* **2013**, *91*, 134–138.
9. Bæk, K.T.; Gründling, A.; Mogensen, R.G.; Thøgersen, L.; Petersen, A.; Paulander, W.; Frees, D. β-Lactam resistance in methicillin-resistant *Staphylococcus aureus* USA300 is increased by inactivation of the ClpXP protease. *Antimicrob. Agents Chemother.* **2014**, *58*, 4593–4603. [CrossRef]
10. Ben Nejma, M.; Mastouri, M.; Bel Hadj Jrad, B.; Nour, M. Characterization of ST80 Panton-Valentine Leukocidin-positive community-acquired methicillin resistant *Staphylococcus aureus* clone in Tunisia. *Diagn. Microbiol. Infect. Dis.* **2013**, *77*, 20–24. [CrossRef]
11. Kechrid, A.; Pérez-Vázquez, M.; Smaoui, H.; Hariga, D.; Rodríguez-Baños, M.; Vindel, A.; Baquero, F.; Cantón, R.; del Campo, R. Molecular Analysis of Community-Acquired Methicillin-Susceptible and Resistant *Staphylococcus aureus* Isolates Recovered from Bacteraemic and Osteomyelitis Infections in Children from Tunisia. *Clin. Microbiol. Infect.* **2011**, *17*, 1020–1026. [CrossRef]
12. Mariem, B.J.J.; Ito, T.; Zhang, M.; Jin, J.; Li, S.; Ilhem, B.-B.B.; Adnan, H.; Han, X.; Hiramatsu, K. Molecular Characterization of Methicillin-Resistant Panton-Valentine Leukocidin positive *Staphylococcus aureus* clones disseminating in Tunisian Hospitals and in the Community. *BMC Microbiol.* **2013**, *13*, 2. [CrossRef] [PubMed]
13. Benouda, A.; Elhamzaui, S. *Staphylococcus aureus*: Epidemiologie et prevalence des souches resistantes a la methicilline (SARM) au Maroc. *Rev. Tunis. D'Infect.* **2009**, *3*, 15–20.
14. Rice, L.B. Mechanisms of Resistance and Clinical Relevance of Resistance to β-Lactams, Glycopeptides, and Fluoroquinolones. *Mayo Clin. Proc.* **2012**, *87*, 198–208. [CrossRef] [PubMed]

15. Falagas, M.E.; Karageorgopoulos, D.E.; Leptidis, J.; Korbila, I.P. MRSA in Africa: Filling the Global Map of Antimicrobial Resistance. *PLoS ONE* **2013**, *8*, e68024. [CrossRef]
16. Baig, S.; Johannesen, T.B.; Overballe-Petersen, S.; Larsen, J.; Larsen, A.R.; Stegger, M. Novel SCC*mec* Type XIII (9A) identified in an ST152 Methicillin-Resistant *Staphylococcus aureus*. *Infect. Genet. Evol.* **2018**, *61*, 74–76. [CrossRef] [PubMed]
17. Zmantar, T.; Kouidhi, B.; Hentati, H.; Bakhrouf, A. Detection of disinfectant and antibiotic resistance genes in *Staphylococcus aureus* isolated from the oral cavity of Tunisian children. *Ann. Microbiol.* **2012**, *62*, 123–128. [CrossRef]
18. Goolam Mahomed, T.; Kock, M.M.; Masekela, R.; Hoosien, E.; Ehlers, M.M. Genetic relatedness of *Staphylococcus aureus* isolates obtained from cystic fibrosis patients at a tertiary academic hospital in Pretoria, South Africa. *Sci. Rep.* **2018**, *8*, 12222. [CrossRef]
19. Jemili-Ben Jomaa, M.; Boutiba-Ben Boubaker, I.; Ben Redjeb, S. Identification of staphylococcal cassette chromosome *mec* encoding methicillin resistance in *Staphylococcus aureus* isolates at Charles Nicolle Hospital of Tunis. *Pathol. Biol.* **2006**, *54*, 453–455. [CrossRef]
20. Bouchami, O.; Achour, A.; Ben Hassan, A. Typing of staphylococcal cassette chromosome *mec* encoding methicillin resistance in *Staphylococcus aureus* strains isolated at the bone marrow transplant centre of Tunisia. *Curr. Microbiol.* **2009**, *59*, 380–385. [CrossRef]
21. Gharsa, H.; Dziri, R.; Klibi, N.; Chairat, S.; Lozano, C.; Torres, C.; Bellaaj, R.; Slama, K.B. Environmental *Staphylococcus aureus* contamination in a Tunisian hospital. *J. Chemother.* **2016**, *28*, 506–509. [CrossRef]
22. Rodrigues, M.V.P.; Fortaleza, C.M.C.B.; Riboli, D.F.M.; Rocha, R.S.; Rocha, C.; de Souza da Cunha, M.d.L.R. Molecular epidemiology of methicillin-resistant *Staphylococcus aureus* in a burn unit from Brazil. *Burns* **2013**, *39*, 1242–1249. [CrossRef] [PubMed]
23. Namvar, A.E.; Afshar, M.; Asghari, B.; Rastegar Lari, A. Characterisation of SCC*mec* elements in methicillin-resistant *Staphylococcus aureus* isolated from burn patients. *Burns* **2014**, *40*, 708–712. [CrossRef]
24. Asadollahi, P.; Farahani, N.N.; Mirzaii, M.; Khoramrooz, S.S.; van Belkum, A.; Asadollahi, K.; Dadashi, M.; Darban-Sarokhalil, D. Distribution of the most prevalent *spa*-types among clinical isolates of methicillin-resistant and susceptible *Staphylococcus aureus* around the world: A Review. *Front. Microbiol.* **2018**, *9*, 163. [CrossRef] [PubMed]
25. Elhani, D.; Gharsa, H.; Kalai, D.; Lozano, C.; Gómez, P.; Boutheina, J.; Aouni, M.; Barguellil, F.; Torres, C.; Ben Slama, K. Clonal lineages detected amongst tetracycline resistant meticillin resistant *Staphylococcus aureus* isolates of a Tunisian hospital, with detection of lineage ST398. *J. Med. Microbiol.* **2015**, *64*, 623–629. [CrossRef] [PubMed]
26. Ikonomidis, A.; Vasdeki, A.; Kristo, I.; Maniatis, A.N.; Tsakris, A.; Malizos, K.N.; Pournaras, S. Association of Biofilm Formation and Methicillin-Resistance with Accessory Gene Regulator (*Agr*) Loci in Greek *Staphylococcus aureus* Clones. *Microb. Pathog.* **2009**, *47*, 341–344. [CrossRef] [PubMed]
27. Holtfreter, S.; Grumann, D.; Schmudde, M.; Nguyen, H.T.T.; Eichler, P.; Strommenger, B.; Kopron, K.; Kolata, J.; Giedrys-Kalemba, S.; Steinmetz, I.; et al. Clonal distribution of superantigen genes in clinical *Staphylococcus aureus* isolates. *J. Clin. Microbiol.* **2007**, *45*, 2669–2680. [CrossRef]
28. Robinson, D.A.; Enright, M.C. Evolutionary models of the emergence of methicillin resistant *Staphylococcus aureus*. *Antimicrob. Agents Chemother.* **2003**, *47*, 3926–3934. [CrossRef]
29. Xu, Y.; Qian, S.-Y.; Yao, K.-H.; Dong, F.; Song, W.-Q.; Sun, C.; Yang, X.; Zhen, J.-H.; Liu, X.-Q.; Lv, Z.-Y.; et al. Clinical and molecular characteristics of *Staphylococcus aureus* isolated from chinese children: Association among the *agr* groups and genotypes, Virulence Genes and Disease Types. *World J. Pediatr.* **2021**, *17*, 180–188. [CrossRef]
30. Dunyach-Remy, C.; Ngba Essebe, C.; Sotto, A.; Lavigne, J.-P. *Staphylococcus aureus* toxins and diabetic foot ulcers: Role in pathogenesis and interest in diagnosis. *Toxins* **2016**, *8*, 209. [CrossRef]
31. Víquez-Molina, G.; Aragón-Sánchez, J.; Pérez-Corrales, C.; Murillo-Vargas, C.; López-Valverde, M.E.; Lipsky, B.A. Virulence factor genes in *Staphylococcus aureus* isolated from diabetic foot soft tissue and bone infections. *Int. J. Low. Extrem. Wounds* **2018**, *17*, 36–41. [CrossRef]
32. Mottola, C.; Semedo-Lemsaddek, T.; Mendes, J.J.; Melo-Cristino, J.; Tavares, L.; Cavaco-Silva, P.; Oliveira, M. Molecular typing, virulence traits and antimicrobial resistance of diabetic foot staphylococci. *J. Biomed. Sci.* **2016**, *23*, 33. [CrossRef] [PubMed]
33. Lina, G.; Piemont, Y.; Godail-Gamot, F.; Bes, M.; Peter, M.-O.; Gauduchon, V.; Vandenesch, F.; Etienne, J. Involvement of Panton-Valentine Leukocidin producing *Staphylococcus aureus* in primary skin infections and pneumonia. *Clin. Infect. Dis.* **1999**, *29*, 1128–1132. [CrossRef] [PubMed]
34. Gillet, Y.; Issartel, B.; Vanhems, P.; Fournet, J.-C.; Lina, G.; Bes, M.; Vandenesch, F.; Piémont, Y.; Brousse, N.; Floret, D.; et al. Association between *Staphylococcus aureus* strains carrying gene for Panton-Valentine Leukocidin and highly lethal necrotising pneumonia in young immunocompetent patients. *Lancet* **2002**, *359*, 753–759. [CrossRef] [PubMed]
35. Brosnahan, A.J.; Schlievert, P.M. Gram-positive bacterial superantigen outside-in signaling causes toxic shock syndrome: Superantigen outside-in signaling. *FEBS J.* **2011**, *278*, 4649–4667. [CrossRef]
36. Budzyńska, A.; Skowron, K.; Kaczmarek, A.; Wietlicka-Piszcz, M.; Gospodarek-Komkowska, E. virulence factor genes and antimicrobial susceptibility of *Staphylococcus aureus* strains isolated from blood and chronic wounds. *Toxins* **2021**, *13*, 491. [CrossRef]
37. Ji, G.; Beavis, R.C.; Novick, R.P. Cell density control of staphylococcal virulence mediated by an octapeptide pheromone. *Proc. Natl. Acad. Sci. USA* **1995**, *92*, 12055–12059. [CrossRef]

38. Sakoulas, G. The cacessory gene regulator (*agr*) in methicillin resistant *Staphylococcus aureus*: Role in virulence and reduced susceptibility to glycopeptide Antibiotics. *Drug. Discov. Today* **2006**, *3*, 287–294. [CrossRef]
39. Klibi, A.; Jouini, A.; Gómez, P.; Slimene, K.; Ceballos, S.; Torres, C.; Maaroufi, A. Molecular characterization and clonal diversity of methicillin resistant and susceptible *Staphylococcus aureus* isolates of milk of cows with clinical mastitis in Tunisia. *Microb. Drug. Resist.* **2018**, *24*, 1210–1216. [CrossRef]
40. Clinical and Laboratory Standards Institute (CLSI). *Performance Standards for Antimicrobial Susceptibility Testing*; Twenty-Fifth Informational Supplement; CLSI document M100-S25: Clinical Laboratory Standard Institute: Wayne, PA, USA, 2015.
41. Zhang, K.; Sparling, J.; Chow, B.L.; Elsayed, S.; Hussain, Z.; Church, D.L.; Gregson, D.B.; Louie, T.; Conly, J.M. New quadriplex PCR assay for detection of methicillin and mupirocin resistance and simultaneous discrimination of *Staphylococcus aureus* from coagulase-negative staphylococci. *J. Clin. Microbiol.* **2004**, *42*, 4947–4955. [CrossRef]
42. Kondo, Y.; Ito, T.; Ma, X.X.; Watanabe, S.; Kreiswirth, B.N.; Etienne, J.; Hiramatsu, K. Combination of multiplex PCRs for staphylococcal cassette chromosome *mec* type assignment: Rapid identification system for *mec*, *ccr* and major differences in junkyard regions. *Antimicrob. Agents Chemother.* **2007**, *51*, 264–274. [CrossRef]
43. Harmsen, D.; Claus, H.; Witte, W.; Rothganger, J.; Claus, H.; Turnwald, D.; Vogel, U. Typing of methicillin-resistant *Staphylococcus aureus* in a university hospital setting by using novel software for *spa* repeat determination and database management. *J. Clin. Microbiol.* **2003**, *41*, 5442–5448. [CrossRef] [PubMed]
44. Shopsin, B.; Mathema, B.; Alcabes, P.; Said-Salim, B.; Lina, G.; Matsuka, A.; Martinez, J.; Kreiswirth, B.N. Prevalence of *agr* specificity groups among *Staphylococcus aureus* strains colonizing children and their guardians. *J. Clin. Microbiol.* **2003**, *41*, 456–459. [CrossRef] [PubMed]
45. Gharsa, H.; Ben Slama, K.; Lozano, C.; Gómez-Sanz, E.; Klibi, N.; Ben Sallem, R.; Gómez, P.; Zarazaga, M.; Boudabous, A.; Torres, C. Prevalence, antibiotic resistance, virulence traits and genetic lineages of *Staphylococcus aureus* in healthy sheep in Tunisia. *Vet. Microbiol.* **2012**, *156*, 367–373. [CrossRef] [PubMed]
46. Hwang, S.Y.; Kim, S.H.; Jang, E.J.; Kwon, N.H.; Park, Y.K.; Koo, H.C.; Jung, W.K.; Kim, J.M.; Park, Y.H. Novel multiplex PCR for the detection of the Staphylococcus aureus superantigen and its application to raw meat isolates in Korea. *Int. J. Food Microbiol.* **2007**, *117*, 99–105. [CrossRef] [PubMed]
47. Van Wamel, W.J.B.; Rooijakkers, S.H.M.; Ruyken, M.; Van Kessel, K.P.M.; Van Strijp, J.A.G. The innate immune modulators staphylococcal complement inhibitor and chemotaxis inhibitory protein of *Staphylococcus aureus* are located on β-hemolysin-converting bacteriophages. *J. Bacteriol.* **2006**, *188*, 1310–1315. [CrossRef]

antibiotics

MDPI

Article

Antimicrobial Resistance of *Staphylococcus aureus* Isolated between 2017 and 2022 from Infections at a Tertiary Care Hospital in Romania

Daniela Tălăpan [1,2,*], Andreea-Mihaela Sandu [2] and Alexandru Rafila [1,2]

1 Microbiology Department I, Faculty of Medicine, "Carol Davila" University of Medicine and Pharmacy, 050474 Bucharest, Romania; andreeasandu30@gmail.com (A.-M.S.); alexandru.rafila@umfcd.ro (A.R.)
2 "Prof. Dr. Matei Balș" National Institute of Infectious Diseases, 021105 Bucharest, Romania
* Correspondence: daniela.talapan@umfcd.ro; Tel.: +0040-723672483

Abstract: This study aimed to evaluate the frequency of isolation of *Staphylococcus aureus* from different pathological samples processed in the Microbiology Laboratory of the National Institute of Infectious Diseases "Prof. Dr. Matei Balș", Romania, between 1 January 2017 and 31 December 2022, aiming to establish the ratio of methicillin-resistant to methicillin-susceptible *Staphylococcus aureus* strains and the antibiotic resistance pattern of isolated microorganisms. The data of isolates originating from routine diagnostic tasks were analyzed retrospectively using laboratory data from the microbiology department. Up to 39.11% of *Staphylococcus aureus* strains were resistant to oxacillin (MRSA), with 49.97% resistance to erythromycin and 36.06% inducible resistance to clindamycin. Resistance rates to ciprofloxacin, rifampicin, gentamicin, and trimethoprim-sulfamethoxazole were 9.98%, 5.38%, 5.95%, and 0.96%, respectively. There was no resistance to vancomycin. Between 2017 and 2022, the percentage of MRSA strains decreased from 41.71% to 33.63%, sharply increasing to 42.42% in 2021 (the year of the COVID-19 pandemic, when the percentage of strains isolated from lower respiratory tract infections was higher than that of strains isolated from wounds or blood, as in previous years). This study showed a high percentage of MRSA strains (39.11% overall) with a higher proportion of these strains isolated from the blood (42.49%) compared to other clinical specimens.

Keywords: resistance; *Staphylococcus aureus*; MRSA; Romania

1. Introduction

Staphylococcus aureus, a Gram-positive bacterium commonly found in the environment, is part of the natural flora of human beings [1]. Most healthy people (over 60%) have this bacterium on their skins and mucous membranes of their upper respiratory tracts, primarily in the nares [2,3]. Approximately 20% of people are long-term carriers [4]. Most of these individuals do not experience any clinical symptoms, as it rarely causes infections if the skin is intact [5]. However, *Staphylococcus aureus* can spread to the bloodstream or internal soft tissues. In that case, it can potentially cause various infectious diseases ranging from minor skin infections and soft tissue infections, such as impetigo, cellulitis, scalded skin syndrome, folliculitis, and abscesses, to severe life-threatening conditions such as fatal pneumonia, osteomyelitis, toxic shock syndrome, endocarditis, and bacteremia [6,7].

It is estimated that infectious diseases are the second most significant cause of mortality globally. The growing danger of drug-resistant microorganisms poses a severe public health problem globally [8]. *Staphylococcus aureus*, which is widely recognized as a significant pathogen in clinical and community environments, is notoriously resistant to penicillin and other antimicrobials [9]. The production of β-lactamase enzymes causes this resistance, with the first report of a penicillin-resistant strain of *Staphylococcus aureus* published in 1945 [10,11]. In 1884, Friedrich Julius Rosenbach first identified this bacterium. However, it was not until the 1930s that enzyme testing was used to detect a staphylococcal infection due to coagulase production by this microorganism. Physicians then began diagnosing and treating *Staphylococcus aureus* using penicillin. Before 1940, 75% of those infected with *Staphylococcus aureus* would die. However, by the end of the 1940s, a resistant strain had developed, causing traditional penicillin to no longer effectively treat the infection [2,12].

The methicillin-resistant *Staphylococcus aureus* (MRSA) is a strain resistant to all penicillin, including methicillin and other narrow-spectrum β-lactamase-resistant penicillin antimicrobials. Moreover, it has been a great challenge to medicine since MRSA causes the same types of infections as other strains of *Staphylococcus aureus* but is resistant to the most common antimicrobials [13]. The rise and dissemination of MRSA, comprising both hospital-associated MRSA (HA-MRSA) and community-associated MRSA (CA-MRSA), is a significant issue on a global scale [14,15]. The emergence of antibiotic resistance in *Staphylococcus aureus* has been attributed mainly to the acquisition of genetic determinants through the horizontal gene transfer of mobile genetic elements [16], the alteration of drug binding sites on molecular targets, and the increased expression of efflux pumps. Conventionally, HA-MRSA has been linked with multidrug resistance and staphylococcal cassette chromosome mec (SCC*mec*) types I, II, and III, while CA-MRSA has been connected to SCC*mec* types IV and V and the presence of Panton-Valentine leukocidin genes. Combinations of inhibitors targeting different sites were used to reduce the probability of resistance arising from mutations [10,14].

Notwithstanding, only some antibiotics with novel chemical classes have been introduced in the past 30 years. Here are some examples of drug classes used to treat *Staphylococcus aureus* infections and their mechanisms of action. Vancomycin, a glycopeptide antibiotic, is extensively used to treat severe infections caused by MRSA strains in hospitalized patients. It binds to the dipeptide D-Ala4-D-Ala5 of lipid II, blocking the transglycosylation and transpeptidation catalyzed by PBP2 (penicillin-binding protein 2) and PBP2a (penicillin-binding protein 2), a protein that is essential to bacterial cell wall synthesis and can prevent peptidoglycan remodeling [9,17]. With vancomycin, up to six gene mutations are required to reduce drug access to the lethal target [10]. Linezolid, an oxazolidinone drug, was approved in the year 2000 for the treatment of challenging HA-MRSA infections. Linezolid is the only wholly synthetic antibiotic that acts on the ribosome. The binding site is in the ribosomal peptidyl transferase center (PTC) in the 50S ribosome subunit, and it impairs the amino-acyl moiety of aa-tRNA, inhibiting peptidyl transferase and peptide bond formation [18,19]. Erythromycin is a macrolide that inhibits the polypeptide exit next to the PTC. Currently, macrolides are not regularly used to treat staphylococcal infections but have a role in *Staphylococcus aureus* infections. Semisynthetic macrolides, such as clarithromycin and azithromycin are used therapeutically to treat bacterial infections caused by microorganisms different from this one. As a result, the commensal staphylococci are regularly exposed to macrolides, which may account for erythromycin resistance being commonly identified in clinical specimens [12,19].

In recent studies, it has been observed that some patients suffering from COVID-19 developed pulmonary bacterial co-infection (identified within 48 h of presentation) and secondary infections (identified after 48 h of admission) or superinfection, which has a negative effect on their prognosis [8,20]. There is considerable variance in the literature regarding the epidemiology of MRSA lung infections in patients with COVID-19, with the relative prevalence ranging from 2% to 29% when all other bacteria are considered and from 11% to 65% when *Staphylococcus aureus* is the common denominator [21,22]. Although various patient-specific environmental factors could be responsible for the predominance of *Staphylococcus aureus* co-infections post-admission in patients with COVID-19, the findings of previous studies suggest that this infection may be partially attributed to the treatment course. Overall, MRSA remains one of the most frequently encountered causative pathogens of pulmonary infections in patients with COVID-19 [20,23–25].

Therefore, in this study, we aimed to evaluate the frequency of isolation of *Staphylococcus aureus* from different pathological samples processed in the Microbiology Laboratory of the National Institute of Infectious Diseases "Prof. Dr. Matei Balș", Romania, between 1

January 2017, and 31 December 2022, to establish the ratio of MRSA strains to methicillin-susceptible *Staphylococcus aureus* strains (MSSA) and the trend in the frequency of isolation of MRSA strains in different clinical specimens and also to monitor the resistance of MRSA/MSSA strains to non-beta-lactam antibiotics.

2. Results

2.1. The Source of Staphylococcus aureus Strains

A total of 1672 *Staphylococcus aureus* strains were isolated between 2017 and 2022, with the numbers per clinical specimen being similar between the pre-pandemic years (2017–2019) and reducing during the COVID-19 pandemic and the post-pandemic years (2020–2022). Staphylococci were most commonly isolated from wounds (57.78%), followed by blood (18.72%), lower respiratory tract secretions (9.39%), ocular secretions (8.01%), and then from the urine, ear secretions, pleural fluid, and joint fluid (6.1%) (Table 1).

Table 1. *Staphylococcus aureus* strains and clinical specimens from which they were isolated.

Year	Wound Secretion (N)	Blood (N)	LRT [a] (N)	Eye Secretion (N)	Other [b] (N)	Total N (%)
2017	245	68	21	45	31	410 (24.52)
2018	237	75	23	33	13	381 (22.79)
2019	276	87	22	31	30	446 (26.67)
2020	54	27	15	6	8	110 (6.58)
2021	25	17	43	4	10	99 (5.92)
2022	129	39	33	15	10	226 (13.52)
Total N (%)	966 (57.78)	313 (18.72)	157 (9.39)	134 (8.01)	102 (6.1)	1672 (100)

[a] LRT, lower respiratory tract (sputum, bronchial aspirates, and bronchoalveolar lavage). [b] Other (ear secretion, urine, pleural fluid, and joint fluid).

Over the years, there was no significant difference in the proportion of *Staphylococcus aureus* strains isolated from various clinical specimens, with one exception: in 2021, these bacteria were isolated the most from the lower respiratory tract (LRT, 43.43%; N = 43), compared to wound secretions (25.25%; N = 25), blood (17.17%; N = 17), ocular secretions (4.04%; N = 4), and other clinical specimens (10.10%; N = 10), p value < 0.001.

2.2. Antimicrobial Susceptibility

A summary of the antimicrobial susceptibility of *Staphylococcus aureus* strains is provided in Figure 1. Up to 39.11% of *Staphylococcus aureus* strains were MRSA, with no strain being resistant to vancomycin but with two of them being resistant to linezolid (0.12%) and three being resistant to teicoplanin (0.18%). The three strains that were resistant to teicoplanin had different minimum inhibitory concentrations (MICs); one had 4 mg/L and two had 8 mg/L, and 18 out of 1672 (1.08%) strains had elevated MIC (2 mg/L). Moreover, 22 out of 1672 (1.32%) strains had vancomycin MIC = 2 mg/L. Among all *Staphylococcus aureus* strains, two were resistant to linezolid (MIC > 4 mg/L), but 17 out of 1672 (1.02%) had a MIC of four, with the rest of them having MICs of $\leq$2.

The rate of resistance to erythromycin was high (49.97%), and the rate of inducible resistance to clindamycin was 36.06%. The lowest resistance rate (<10%) was that of resistance to ciprofloxacin, moxifloxacin, gentamycin, rifampicin, and trimethoprim-sulfamethoxazole.

The rate of penicillin resistance was high in all strains (>80%), regardless of the clinical specimen (Figure 2). MRSA strains were most commonly isolated from the blood (oxacillin resistance: 42.49%), followed by wound secretions (39.85%) and the lower respiratory tract (37.13%), and, to a lesser extent, from other clinical specimens (ear secretions, urine, pleural fluid, and joint fluid, 29.41%; ocular secretions, 23.88%). *Staphylococcus aureus* strains isolated from ocular secretions were less resistant to all antimicrobials compared to the strains isolated from other clinical specimens, except for gentamicin, where resistance was similar for the strains isolated from wound secretions.

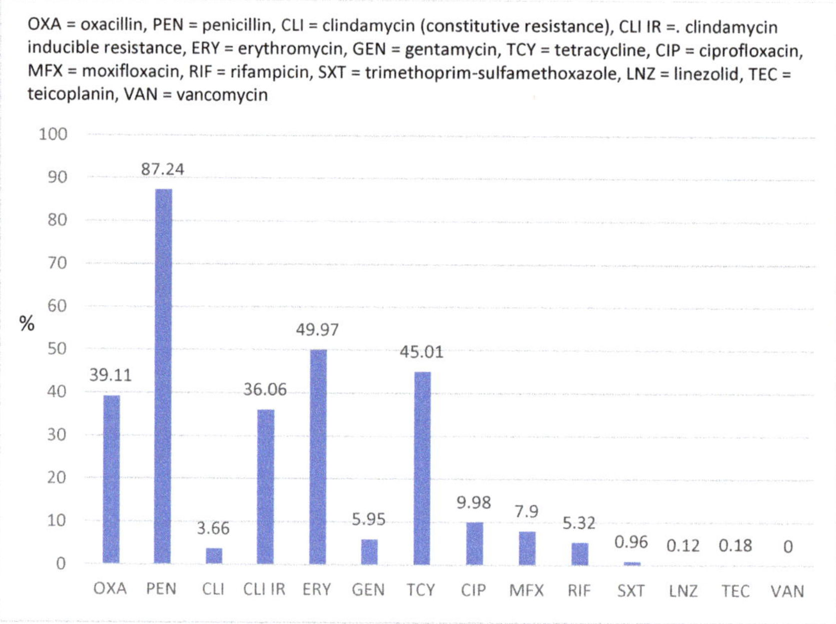

Figure 1. Overall rates of resistance to antimicrobials of *Staphylococcus aureus* strains (N = 1672) isolated between 2017 and 2022.

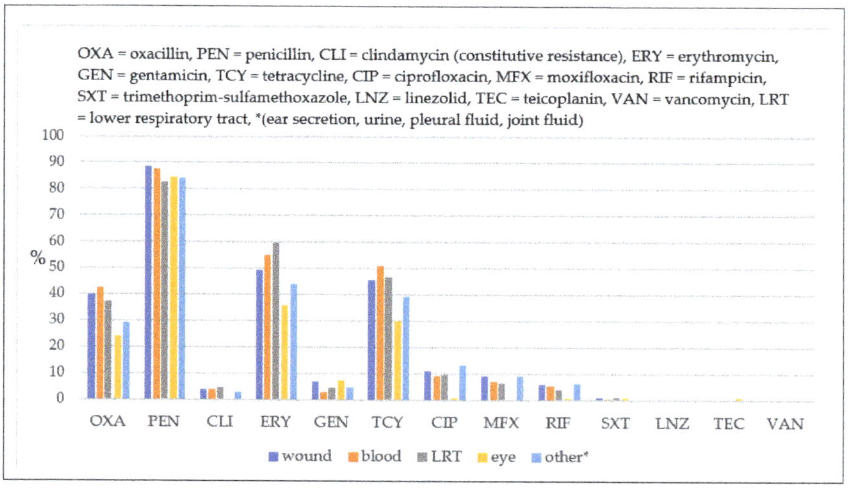

Figure 2. Comparative resistance of *Staphylococcus aureus* strains isolated from different clinical specimens.

MRSA strains varied over the years (Figure 3), having a steady decrease from 2017 (41.71%) to 2022 (33.63%), with a sharp and significant increase in 2021 compared to 2020 (42.63% vs. 35.35%, $p < 0.001$).

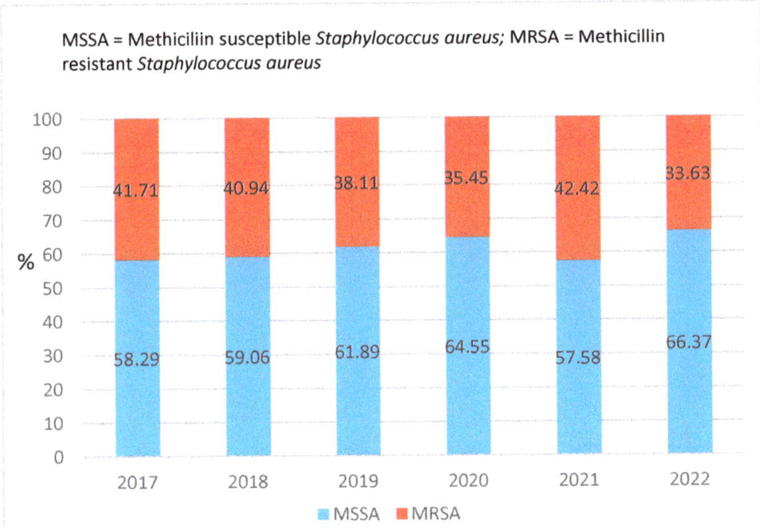

Figure 3. MRSA evolution between 2017 and 2022.

MRSA strains were more resistant to all antimicrobials than MSSA strains (Figure 4) with one exception: linezolid, to which only two MSSA strains were resistant (0.2%). None of the strains were resistant to vancomycin.

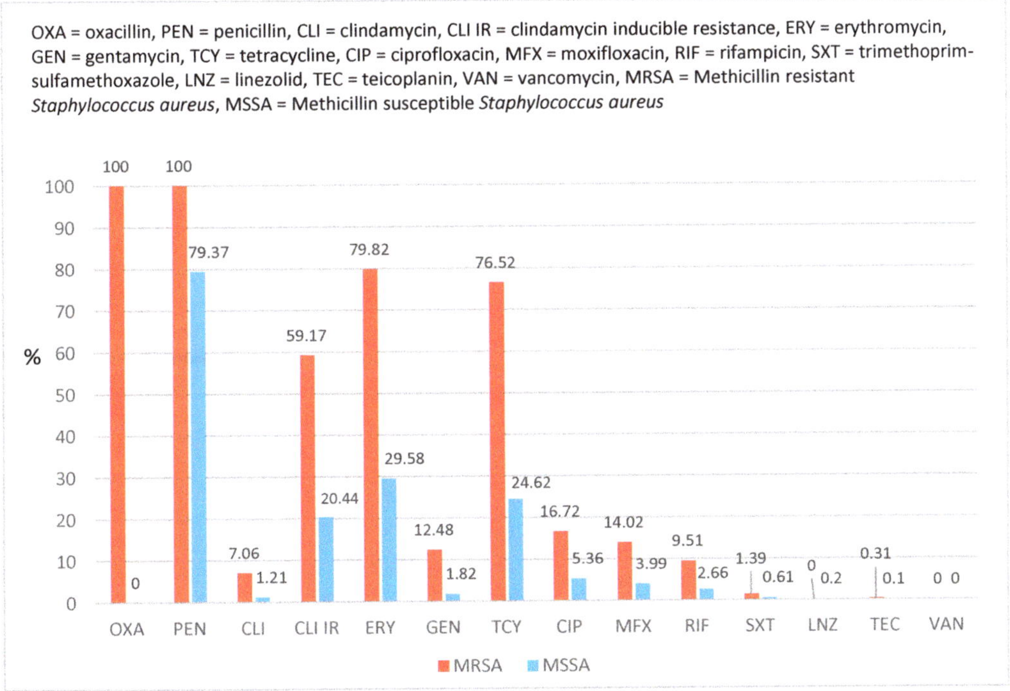

Figure 4. Comparative resistance between methicillin-resistant and methicillin-susceptible *Staphylococcus aureus* strains.

MRSA strains showed an increased resistance rate to tetracycline in 2022 compared to 2017 (48.26% vs. 70.27%, $p = 0.09$), fluoroquinolones (ciprofloxacin 10.47% vs. 16.88%, $p = 0.21$; moxifloxacin 6.98% vs. 18.42%, $p = 0.01$), and rifampicin (6.4% vs. 18.42%, $p = 0.06$) (Figure 5); however, the increase was not statistically significant. Decreased resistance to clindamycin (from 83.23% in 2017 to 56.96% in 2022, $p = 0.88$) and erythromycin (from 83.14% to 73.42%, $p = 0.54$) was observed. Resistance to gentamicin and trimethoprim-sulfamethoxazole remained low and variable through the years.

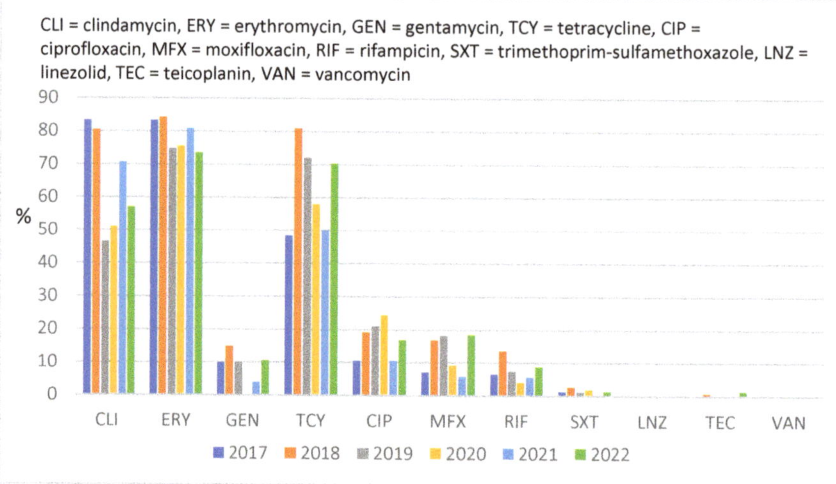

Figure 5. Resistance to non-beta-lactam antimicrobials of MRSA strains isolated between 2017 and 2022.

3. Discussion

In the CDC's antibiotic resistance threats report from 2019, MRSA was placed in the "serious threats-public health threats that require prompt and sustained action" category, being responsible for approximately 323,700 infections in hospitalized patients, with an estimated 10,600 deaths in 2017 [26]. In Europe, between 2017 and 2019, the MRSA rate among invasive infections in the European Union according to the European Centre for Disease Prevention and Control antimicrobial resistance surveillance found Romania on top of the list, with 45.4%, 43%, and 46.9%, respectively. Only in 2020 was Romania in second place (after Cyprus, 49.1%) despite having an even higher rate than the previous one (47.3%). In 2021, Romania came third with 41% (after Cyprus, 42.9% and Greece, 41.9%) [27]. Several previous studies have reported the rates of MRSA infections in Romania to range from approximately 30% to 70% [28–33].

This study presents evidence of *Staphylococcus aureus* resistance to different antimicrobial agents. Bacterial strains were isolated from samples obtained from infected patients in a tertiary mono-disciplinary hospital, which was declared a COVID-19-dedicated hospital and attended only to patients who tested positive for SARS-CoV-2 virus either by PCR (polymerase chain reaction) or antigen detection in the nasopharyngeal swab from March 2020 to May 2022. From 2017 through 2022, 1672 strains of *Staphylococcus aureus* were isolated. The number of strains isolated during the pre-pandemic years (2017–2019) was higher than those isolated during the COVID-19 pandemic and post-pandemic years (2020–2022). There was no significant distinction in the percentage of isolated strains from different clinical samples, except in 2021 when most isolations were from the lower respiratory tract (43.43%). Our results are similar to those presented by De Santis et al., according to which *Staphylococcus aureus* was most commonly isolated from respiratory samples of patients with COVID-19 (31.1%) [34].

The report summarizes the antimicrobial susceptibility of *Staphylococcus aureus* strains. Approximately 39% of the strains were shown to be MRSA, and no resistance to vancomycin was detected, perhaps because vancomycin treatment in eligible patients in Romania is performed only in the hospital over a short course of two weeks. However, a small percent of strains (22 out of 1672; 1.32%) had vancomycin MIC = 2 mg/L, which is on the border of the wild-type distribution and may be an impaired clinical response if used, according to the European Committee on Antimicrobial Susceptibility Testing (EUCAST) guidelines. It had been feared that MRSA might acquire vancomycin (Van) resistance from enterococci, resulting in untreatable invasive severe infection. Although there have been a few isolated cases of vancomycin-resistant *Staphylococcus aureus* (VRSA), these strains have not spread and have not become a permanent presence in hospitals [35,36].

Two other strains (0.12%) were resistant to linezolid, and three (0.18%) were resistant to teicoplanin. Staphylococcal isolates with reduced susceptibility to glycopeptides, such as vancomycin and teicoplanin, are a significant public health concern because staphylococci are often resistant to various drugs. Glycopeptides are widely used in Europe, where vancomycin is the antibiotic of choice for treating MRSA infections; however, in cases such as endocarditis, osteomyelitis, and septic arthritis, teicoplanin could be considered [37]. Since glycopeptides may be the only remaining effective drugs, initial reports of glycopeptide-resistant staphylococci have caused alarm [38]. The development of resistance to teicoplanin has been documented in cases of MRSA [39]. There have been reports in the literature of MRSA strains that are resistant to teicoplanin but susceptible to vancomycin. Both in vitro and in vivo studies have demonstrated that the MIC of teicoplanin increased 2–16 times; whereas, those for vancomycin only increased by less than two times [37,39,40]. Another study by Majchrzak et al. showed that out of the 600 MRSA strains, 47 (representing 7.83%) were glycopeptide-resistant, and 11 (23.4%) were confirmed to be VRSA. In contrast, the remaining 36 (76.6%) were shown to be resistant only to teicoplanin [41]. Our study also found that out of all *Staphylococcus aureus* strains, only 3 (0.18%) exhibited resistance to teicoplanin, while none exhibited resistance to vancomycin. Teicoplanin resistance has become more prevalent than vancomycin resistance since the initial reports of glycopeptide-resistant staphylococci [42].

Considerable resistance to erythromycin (49.97%) was observed, and the rate of clindamycin-inducible resistance was 36.06%. Ciprofloxacin, moxifloxacin, gentamicin, rifampicin, and trimethoprim-sulfamethoxazole had the lowest resistance rates (all <10%). MRSA strains have experienced a general decline from 2017 (41.71%) to 2022 (33.63%), with a notable spike in 2021 (42.63%), the second year of the COVID-19 pandemic. Moreover, the rate of bacterial secondary infection in patients hospitalized for COVID-19 was high worldwide. In a study conducted in Medellin, Columbia, *Staphylococcus aureus* was the second most isolated microorganism (24%), and in another study conducted in Italy, 40.7% of patients were co-infected with it [36,43]. Per our findings, in 2021, this bacterium was most commonly isolated from the lower respiratory tract (43.43%).

Despite originating from the bacterium, the two strains of *Staphylococcus aureus* (methicillin-resistant and methicillin-susceptible) have distinct resistance and virulence factors, which contribute to determining the type of population affected, their capability to combat traditional treatment methods, and their overall rate of mortality and morbidity [19]. The MRSA strains isolated in this study were more resistant to antimicrobials than the MSSA ones, with the sole exception of linezolid, for which only two MSSA strains (0.2%) were resistant. When introducing linezolid, they asserted it would not be subject to cross-resistance and that resistance would hardly develop. However, evidence of resistance has emerged [20]. There appears to be a correlation between the clinical use of linezolid and a decrease in the MIC of vancomycin in *Staphylococcus aureus*, suggesting that alterations in the clinical application of antibiotics may have an impact on bacterial resistance trends [44].

The rate of penicillin resistance was high in all specimens selected (over 80% of the strains isolated). We found the highest rate of MRSA in blood samples (42.49%), followed by wound secretions (39.85%), the lower respiratory tract (37.13%), and less resistance in the other clinical specimens (such as ear secretions, urine, pleural fluid, and joint fluid—29.41%; ocular secretions—23.88%). *Staphylococcus aureus* strains isolated from ocular secretions had lower resistance to all antimicrobials than those isolated from other specimens, except for gentamycin, for which the resistance was similar to that of the strains isolated from wound secretions. Per the findings of other studies, compared to wound secretions, MSSA-related ocular secretions could be easily cured with regular antibiotics such as erythromycin. Zheng XY et al. observed a correlation between the patient's age and erythromycin resistance, with topical erythromycin being the most popular over-the-counter antimicrobial drug for common childhood illnesses such as conjunctivitis and bacterial dermatitis [45]. We can attribute an increase in antimicrobial resistance to the misuse of antibiotics (non-prescribed use), incorrect dosage, incorrect duration of treatment, or their use to treat non-bacterial diseases.

In conclusion, it is still possible to effectively treat most *Staphylococcus aureus* infections caused by MRSA by switching drugs or using different combinations. However, it should be noted that the treatment of persistent infections, such as infective endocarditis, is difficult because underlying health conditions weaken the immune system and also because bacteria develop the ability to avoid antibiotics by forming biofilms.

4. Materials and Methods

4.1. Study Design and Study Setting

This is a retrospective study conducted between 1 January 2017 and 31 December 2022, at the National Institute of Infectious Diseases "Prof. Dr. Matei Balș" in Bucharest, Romania. This facility is a mono-disciplinary tertiary care hospital, which was a COVID-19-dedicated hospital between March 2020 and mid-2022. The study was conducted per the ethical standards of the 1964 Declaration of Helsinki and its later amendments. The institutional review board of the National Institute of Infectious Diseases "Prof. Dr. Matei Balș" granted access to the data without the need for individual informed consent since the data were to be analyzed anonymously. The data were extracted from the hospital's Microbiology laboratory database.

4.2. Bacterial Culture

Between 2017 and 2022, 1672 non-duplicate strains of *Staphylococcus aureus* were isolated from various clinical specimens collected from patients admitted to this institution. Wound secretions, ocular secretions, and ear secretions were collected with sterile cotton swabs. From the lower respiratory tract, sputum, bronchial aspirates, or bronchoalveolar lavage fluid were collected. *Staphylococcus aureus* strains were also isolated from blood, urine, pleural fluid, and joint fluid.

All clinical specimens were sent immediately to the Microbiology laboratory, which works 24/7, for processing. In the laboratory, Gram smears and cultures on appropriate bacterial growth media–Columbia agar with sheep blood (ThermoFisher Scientific™-Oxoid, Wesel, Germany), chocolate agar Polivitex (bioMérieux S.A., Marcy-l'Etoile, France), and lactose agar (CLED, ThermoFisher Scientific™-Oxoid, Wesel, Germany), were performed per the laboratory procedures. Blood culture bottles (bioMérieux FA Plus, FN Plus, SA, SN, and PF plus, bioMérieux S.A., Marcy-l'Etoile, France) were incubated at 37 °C, and those that tested positive per the BacT/Alert (bioMérieux, Inc., Durham, NC, USA) were removed and processed on a 24/7 basis by performing Gram staining and culture on Columbia sheep blood agar, chocolate agar, and lactose agar.

Plates were incubated in aerobic atmospheres at 35 °C ± 1 °C. Growth was observed at 18–24 h.

4.3. *Staphylococcus aureus* Identification

Staphylococcus aureus strains were identified using Matrix-Assisted Laser Desorption Ionization Time-of-Flight mass spectrometry (MALDI-TOF MS), which detects bacterial proteins in whole-cell extracts. Bacterial spectra were analyzed using the Biotyper®software version 3.1 (Bruker Daltonik GmbH, Bremen, Germany).

4.4. Antimicrobial Susceptibility Testing

Antimicrobial susceptibility testing (AST) was performed per the EUCAST guideline [46]. MICs were detected using the Sensititre™ system (Thermo Scientific™, Cleveland OH, USA) between 2017 and 2018 and using Romania GP 1, GP 2, and GP 3 EUCAST Micronaut plates (Bruker Daltonics GmbH & Co, KG Bremen, Germany) from 2019 to date (Romania GP 1, 2, and 3 EUCAST cards template are presented in Supplementary Material Tables S1–S3 and changes in plates from the previous version are marked in bold). Vitek®AST-P592 cards–see Supplementary Material Table S4 for the template–(bioMérieux SA, Marcy-l'Etoile, France) were also used through the years if the other system was not available. All plates and cards were used per the manufacturer's instructions. Antimicrobials tested included oxacillin, penicillin, clindamycin, erythromycin, gentamycin, tetracycline, ciprofloxacin, moxifloxacin, rifampicin, trimethoprim-sulfamethoxazole, linezolid, teicoplanin, and vancomycin.

If there were *Staphylococcus aureus* strains with resistance to teicoplanin or vancomycin, the broth microdilution method using Micronaut's Vancomycin/Teicoplanin MIC-Strip (MERLIN Diagnostika GmbH, Bornheim-Hersel, Germany) was used to verify the result and find the exact MIC of the strain (Table 2).

Table 2. Vancomycin/Teicoplanin MIC-Strip.

1	2	3	4	5	6	7	8	9	10	11	12
GC	VAN 0.25	VAN 0.5	VAN 1	VAN 2	VAN 4	TEC 0.25	TEC 0.5	TEC 1	TEC 2	TEC 4	TEC 8

GC, Growth Control; VAN, vancomycin; TEC, teicoplanin.

The results were interpreted according to EUCAST breakpoint tables for the interpretation of MICs and zone diameters available for each year (version 7.1 to version 12.0) [47]. The breakpoints changed in time for some of the antimicrobials tested: ciprofloxacin (susceptibility breakpoint changed in 2020 to ≤0.001 mg/L, from ≤1 mg/L in 2019), gentamicin (resistance breakpoint changed in 2022 to >2 mg/L, from >1 mg/L in 2021), and rifampicin (resistance breakpoint changed in 2022 to >0.06 mg/L, from >0.5 mg/L in 2021).

Methicillin/oxacillin resistance was detected phenotypically by determining the MIC determination of oxacillin (if >2 mg/L, then are methicillin-resistant) [47] and by the identification of PBP2a via the Penicillin-Binding Protein (PBP2′) latex agglutination test (PBP2′ TEST KIT, Oxoid Limited, Wade Road, Basingstoke, UK) per EUCAST guidelines for the detection of resistance mechanisms [48].

4.5. Quality Control

Quality control for AST was performed each time when a lot of Micronaut plates, Vitek®AST P592 cards, or Micronaut's Vancomycin/Teicoplanin MIC-Strip was changed, with the *Staphylococcus aureus* ATCC 29213 strain, per the manufacturer's package insert and EUCAST guidelines for internal quality control [49]. The quality control for the PBP2′ TEST KIT was performed per the manufacturer recommendations (for each new lot and weekly thereafter), with a known MSSA (*Staphylococcus aureus* ATCC 292130) and MRSA strain (*Staphylococcus aureus* NCTC 12493–*mec*A positive [49]).

4.6. Data Analysis

If *Staphylococcus aureus* strains were isolated from more than one clinical specimen from the same patient, the invasive strains were kept and the ones that caused local infections were eliminated from the analysis to have non-duplicate strains. Data analysis was performed using Microsoft Excel version 16.66.1 (2022 ©Microsoft). The Chi-square test was used to compare population proportions, and results with a p value of <0.01 were considered statistically significant. All p values were two-tailed.

5. Conclusions

This study demonstrated a high rate of MRSA (39.11% overall), with a higher rate in strains isolated from the blood (42.49%) than in strains isolated from other clinical specimens. With no resistance to vancomycin, we are still confident that infections caused by these bacteria can be treated, even if resistance can emerge, as it happened to teicoplanin and linezolid. While the production of newer drugs is plausible, the implementation of better stewardship practices that may prolong their activity, and more judicious utilization should ensure the continued treatment of many MRSA infections. It is essential to investigate further to maximize clinical treatment results and discover the elements that lead to resistance such as high-risk strains and the molecular genetic makeup responsible for resistance.

Supplementary Materials: The following supporting information can be downloaded at https://www.mdpi.com/article/10.3390/antibiotics12060974/s1, Table S1. Romania GP 1 EUCAST, Table S2. Romania GP 2 EUCAST, Table S3. Romania GP 3 EUCAST, Table S4. VITEK AST-P592 Card.

Author Contributions: Conceptualization: D.T. and A.R.; methodology: D.T.; software: D.T. and A.-M.S.; validation: D.T., A.-M.S. and A.R.; formal analysis: D.T.; investigation: D.T., A.-M.S.; resources: A.R.; data curation: D.T.; writing—original draft preparation: D.T. and A.-M.S.; writing—review and editing: D.T.; visualization: D.T.; A.-M.S. and A.R.; supervision: A.R.; project administration: D.T., A.-M.S. and A.R. All authors have read and agreed to the published version of the manuscript.

Funding: The authors received no external funding for this study.

Institutional Review Board Statement: This study was approved by the Bioethics committee of the National Institute of Infectious Diseases "Prof. Dr. Matei Balş" (reference number: C02920/07.03.2023).

Informed Consent Statement: Not applicable.

Data Availability Statement: Data are available upon reasonable request to the corresponding author.

Conflicts of Interest: The authors declare no conflict of interest.

Abbreviation

MRSA	Methicillin Resistant *Staphylococcus aureus*
MSSA	Methicillin Susceptible *Staphylococcus aureus*
MIC	Minimum Inhibitory Concentration
AST	Antimicrobial Susceptibility Testing
PBP	Penicillin Binding Protein
EUCAST	European Committee on Antimicrobial Susceptibility Testing

References

1. Chambers, H.F.; DeLeo, F.R. Waves of resistance: Staphylococcus aureus in the antibiotic era. *Nat. Rev. Microbiol.* **2009**, *7*, 629–641. [CrossRef]
2. Tsouklidis, N.; Kumar, R.; Heindl, S.E.; Soni, R.; Khan, S. Understanding the Fight Against Resistance: Hospital-Acquired Methicillin-Resistant *Staphylococcus aureus* vs. Community-Acquired Methicillin-Resistant *Staphylococcus aureus*. *Cureus* **2020**, *12*, e8867. [CrossRef]
3. Onyeka, F.I.; Nwobodo, D.; Umenne, I.C.; Atada, E.E.; Ojukwu, C.A.; Aniekwe, M.A.; Philomena, J.J.; Ikem, J.C. Antibiotic Resistance Pattern of *Staphylococcus aureus* Isolated from Nostrils of Healthy Undergraduates of Madonna University Elele Campus, Rivers State, Nigeria. *Microbes Infect. Dis.* **2020**, *2*, 280–285. [CrossRef]
4. Kluytmans, J.; van Belkum, A.; Verbrugh, H. Nasal carriage of *Staphylococcus aureus*: Epidemiology, underlying mechanisms, and associated risks. *Clin. Microbiol. Rev.* **1997**, *10*, 505–520. [CrossRef]

5. Saba, C.K.S.; Amenyona, J.K.; Kpordze, S.W. Prevalence and pattern of antibiotic resistance of *Staphylococcus aureus* isolated from door handles and other points of contact in public hospitals in Ghana. *Antimicrob. Resist. Infect. Control.* **2017**, *6*, 44. [CrossRef] [PubMed]
6. Lindberg, E.; Adlerberth, I.; Wold, A. Antibiotic resistance in *Staphylococcus aureus* colonising the intestines of Swedish infants. *Clin. Microbiol. Infect.* **2004**, *10*, 890–894. [CrossRef]
7. Gurung, R.R.; Maharjan, P.; Chhetri, G.G. Antibiotic resistance pattern of *Staphylococcus aureus* with reference to MRSA isolates from pediatric patients. *Futur. Sci. OA* **2020**, *6*, FSO464. [CrossRef]
8. CDC. *COVID-19: U.S. Impact on Antimicrobial Resistance, Special Report 2022*; Center for Disease Control and Prevention (CDC): Atlanta, GA, USA, 2022; 1–42. [CrossRef]
9. Akya, A.; Lorestani, R.C.; Shahveisi-Zadeh, J.; Bozorgomid, A. Antimicrobial Resistance of *Staphylococcus aureus* Isolated from Hospital Wastewater in Kermanshah, Iran. *Risk Manag. Health Policy* **2020**, *13*, 1035–1042. [CrossRef] [PubMed]
10. Willis, J.A.; Cheburkanov, V.; Chen, S.; Soares, J.M.; Kassab, G.; Blanco, K.C.; Bagnato, V.S.; de Figueiredo, P.; Yakovlev, V.V. Breaking down antibiotic resistance in methicillin-resistant *Staphylococcus aureus*: Combining antimicrobial photodynamic and antibiotic treatments. *Proc. Natl. Acad. Sci. USA* **2022**, *119*, e2208378119. [CrossRef]
11. Schito, G.C. The importance of the development of antibiotic resistance in *Staphylococcus aureus*. *Clin. Microbiol. Infect.* **2006**, *12*, 3–8. [CrossRef]
12. Arenz, S.; Wilson, D. Blast from the Past: Reassessing Forgotten Translation Inhibitors, Antibiotic Selectivity, and Resistance Mechanisms to Aid Drug Development. *Mol. Cell* **2016**, *61*, 3–14. [CrossRef] [PubMed]
13. Deyno, S.; Toma, A.; Worku, M.; Bekele, M. Antimicrobial resistance profile of *Staphylococcus aureus* isolates isolated from ear discharges of patients at University of Hawassa comprehensive specialized hospital. *BMC Pharmacol. Toxicol.* **2017**, *18*, 1–7. [CrossRef] [PubMed]
14. Santosaningsih, D.; Santoso, S.; Budayanti, N.S.; Suata, K.; Lestari, E.S.; Wahjono, H.; Djamal, A.; Kuntaman, K.; van Belkum, A.; Laurens, M.; et al. Characterisation of clinical *Staphylococcus aureus* isolates harbouring *mecA* or Panton-Valentine leukocidin genes from four tertiary care hospitals in Indonesia. *Trop. Med. Int. Health* **2016**, *21*, 610–618. [CrossRef]
15. Paterson, G.K.; Harrison, E.M.; Holmes, M.A. The emergence of mecC methicillin-resistant *Staphylococcus aureus*. *Trends Microbiol.* **2013**, *22*, 42–47. [CrossRef]
16. Mlynarczyk-Bonikowska, B.; Kowalewski, C.; Krolak-Ulinska, A.; Marusza, W. Molecular Mechanisms of Drug Resistance in *Staphylococcus aureus*. *Int. J. Mol. Sci.* **2022**, *23*, 8088. [CrossRef]
17. Zeng, D.; Debabov, D.; Hartsell, T.L.; Cano, R.J.; Adams, S.; Schuyler, J.A.; McMillan, R.; Pace, J.L. Approved Glycopeptide Antibacterial Drugs: Mechanism of Action and Resistance. *Cold Spring Harb. Perspect. Med.* **2016**, *6*, a026989. [CrossRef] [PubMed]
18. Long, K.S.; Vester, B. Resistance to Linezolid Caused by Modifications at Its Binding Site on the Ribosome. *Antimicrob. Agents Chemother.* **2012**, *56*, 603–612. [CrossRef]
19. Zhou, D.; Steitz, T.A.; Polikanov, Y.S.; Gagnon, M.G. Ribosome-Targeting Antibiotics: Modes of Action, Mechanisms of Resistance, and Implications for Drug Design. *Annu. Rev. Biochem.* **2018**, *87*, 451–478. [CrossRef]
20. Bassetti, M.; Magnasco, L.; Vena, A.; Portunato, F.; Giacobbe, D.R. Methicillin-resistant *Staphylococcus aureus* lung infection in coronavirus disease 2019: How common? *Curr. Opin. Infect. Dis.* **2022**, *35*, 149–162. [CrossRef]
21. Alshaikh, F.S.; Godman, B.; Sindi, O.N.; Seaton, R.A.; Kurdi, A. Prevalence of bacterial coinfection and patterns of antibiotics prescribing in patients with COVID-19: A systematic review and meta-analysis. *PLoS ONE* **2022**, *17*, e0272375. [CrossRef]
22. Arientová, S.; Jícha, Z.; Beran, O.; Holub, M. Decreased quality of care for *Staphylococcus aureus* bacteremia during the COVID-19 pandemic. *BMC Infect. Dis.* **2022**, *22*, 1–5. [CrossRef] [PubMed]
23. O'Toole, R.F. The interface between COVID-19 and bacterial healthcare-associated infections. *Clin. Microbiol. Infect.* **2021**, *27*, 1772–1776. [CrossRef]
24. Adalbert, J.R.; Varshney, K.; Tobin, R.; Pajaro, R. Clinical outcomes in patients co-infected with COVID-19 and *Staphylococcus aureus*: A scoping review. *BMC Infect. Dis.* **2021**, *21*, 1–17. [CrossRef] [PubMed]
25. Habib, G.; Mahmood, K.; Gul, H.; Tariq, M.; Ain, Q.U.; Hayat, A.; Rehman, M.U. Pathophysiology of Methicillin-Resistant *Staphylococcus aureus* Superinfection in COVID-19 Patients. *Pathophysiology* **2022**, *29*, 405–413. [CrossRef]
26. CDC. *Antibiotic Resistance Threats in the United States*; Center for Disease Control and Prevention (CDC): Atlanta, GA, USA, 2019; pp. 1–140. [CrossRef]
27. European Centre for Disease Prevention and Control. Surveillance Atlas of Infectious Diseases. Available online: http://atlas.ecdc.europa.eu/public/index.aspx (accessed on 4 April 2023).
28. Dorneanu, O.; Miftode, E.; Vremeră, T.; Năstase, E.; Filip, O.; Luca, V. Prevalence and characteristics of *Staphylococcus aureus* isolated from infections in Northeast Romania. *J. Prev. Med.* **2006**, *14*, 66–70.
29. Szekely, E.; Lőrinczi, L.; Bilca, D.; Fodor, E.; Soki, J.; Sabau, M. Incidence, antibiotic resistance and clonal relations of MRSA strains isolated from a Romanian university hospital. *Acta Microbiol. et Immunol. Hung.* **2008**, *55*, 1–13. [CrossRef]
30. Ionescu, R.; Mediavilla, J.R.; Chen, L.; Grigorescu, D.O.; Idomir, M.; Kreiswirth, B.N.; Roberts, R.B. Molecular Characterization and Antibiotic Susceptibility of *Staphylococcus aureus* from a Multidisciplinary Hospital in Romania. *Microb. Drug Resist.* **2010**, *16*, 263–272. [CrossRef]

31. Nica, M.; Biolan, T.; Dascalu, A.; Mozes, E.; Toderan, A.; Calistru, P.; Ceauşu, E. Bacterial strains isolated from systemic infections and reported for evaluation and antibiotic resistance surveillance by the "Dr. Victor Babes" Clinical Hospital for Infectious and Tropical Diseases, Bucharest. *Bacteriol. Virusol. Parazitol. Epidemiol.* **2010**, *55*, 161–168.
32. Dorobăţ, O.M.; Bădicuţ, I.; Tălăpan, D.; Tenea, C.; Rafila, A. Antibiotic resistance of Gram-positive cocci isolated in 2008. *Bacteriol. Virusol. Parazitol. Epidemiol.* **2011**, *55*, 83–92.
33. Nastase, E.; Dorneanu, O.; Vremera, T.; Logigan, C.; Miftode, E.; Dorobăţ, C.M. MecA and pvl genes detection in *Staphylococcus aureus* strains isolated from lower respiratory tract infections. *Rev. Med. Chir. Soc. Med. Nat. Iasi.* **2010**, *114*, 1162–1168.
34. De Santis, V.; Corona, A.; Vitale, D.; Nencini, C.; Potalivo, A.; Prete, A.; Zani, G.; Malfatto, A.; Tritapepe, L.; Taddei, S.; et al. Bacterial infections in critically ill patients with SARS-2-COVID-19 infection: Results of a prospective observational multicenter study. *Infection* **2021**, *50*, 139–148. [CrossRef]
35. Gardete, S.; Tomasz, A. Mechanisms of vancomycin resistance in *Staphylococcus* aureus. *J. Clin. Investig.* **2014**, *124*, 2836–2840. [CrossRef]
36. Foster, T.J. Antibiotic resistance in *Staphylococcus aureus.* Current status and future prospects. *FEMS Microbiol. Rev.* **2017**, *41*, 430–449. [CrossRef]
37. Bakthavatchalam, Y.D.; Babu, P.; Munusamy, E.; Dwarakanathan, H.T.; Rupali, P.; Zervos, M.; Victor, P.J.; Veeraraghavan, B. Genomic insights on heterogeneous resistance to vancomycin and teicoplanin in Methicillin-resistant *Staphylococcus aureus*: A first report from South India. *PLoS ONE* **2019**, *14*, e0227009. [CrossRef] [PubMed]
38. Cepeda, J.; Hayman, S.; Whitehouse, T.; Kibbler, C.C.; Livermore, D.; Singer, M.; Wilson, A.P.R. Teicoplanin resistance in methicillin-resistant *Staphylococcus aureus* in an intensive care unit. *J. Antimicrob. Chemother.* **2003**, *52*, 533–534. [CrossRef]
39. McCallum, N.; Karauzum, H.; Getzmann, R.; Bischoff, M.; Majcherczyk, P.; Berger-Bächi, B.; Landmann, R. In Vivo Survival of Teicoplanin-Resistant *Staphylococcus aureus* and Fitness Cost of Teicoplanin Resistance. *Antimicrob. Agents Chemother.* **2006**, *50*, 2352–2360. [CrossRef] [PubMed]
40. Vaudaux, P.; Francois, P.; Berger-Bächi, B.; Lew, D.P. In vivo emergence of subpopulations expressing teicoplanin or vancomycin resistance phenotypes in a glycopeptide-susceptible, methicillin-resistant strain of *Staphylococcus aureus*. *J. Antimicrob. Chemother.* **2001**, *47*, 163–170. [CrossRef] [PubMed]
41. Szymanek-Majchrzak, K.; Mlynarczyk, A.; Mlynarczyk, G. Characteristics of glycopeptide-resistant *Staphylococcus aureus* strains isolated from inpatients of three teaching hospitals in Warsaw, Poland. *Antimicrob. Resist. Infect. Control.* **2018**, *7*, 105. [CrossRef] [PubMed]
42. Tsakris, A.; Papadimitriou, E.; Douboyas, J.; Stylianopoulou, F.; Manolis, E. Emergence of Vancomycin-Intermediate *Staphylococcus aureus* and *S. sciuri*, Greece. *Emerg. Infect. Dis.* **2002**, *8*, 536–537. [CrossRef]
43. Cataño-Correa, J.C.; Cardona-Arias, J.A.; Mancilla, J.P.P.; García, M.T. Bacterial superinfection in adults with COVID-19 hospitalized in two clinics in Medellín-Colombia, 2020. *PLoS ONE* **2021**, *16*, e0254671. [CrossRef]
44. Jian, Y.; Lv, H.; Liu, J.; Huang, Q.; Liu, Y.; Liu, Q.; Li, M. Dynamic Changes of *Staphylococcus aureus* Susceptibility to Vancomycin, Teicoplanin, and Linezolid in a Central Teaching Hospital in Shanghai, China, 2008–2018. *Front. Microbiol.* **2020**, *11*, 908. [CrossRef] [PubMed]
45. Zheng, X.-Y.; Choy, B.N.K.; Zhou, M.-M.; Zhao, Z.-Y. Antibiotic Resistance Pattern of *Staphylococcus aureus* Isolated from Pediatrics with Ocular Infections: A 6-Year Hospital-Based Study in China. *Front. Pediatr.* **2021**, *9*, 728634. [CrossRef] [PubMed]
46. The European Committee on Antimicrobial Susceptibility Testing. Available online: https://www.eucast.org/ast_of_bacteria (accessed on 23 November 2022).
47. The European Committee on Antimicrobial Susceptibility Testing. Breakpoint tables for interpretation of MICs and zone diameters. EUCAST, versions 7.1–12.0, 2017–2022. Available online: https://www.eucast.org/ast_of_bacteria/previous_versions_of_documents/ (accessed on 21 February 2023).
48. The European Committee on Antimicrobial Susceptibility Testing. EUCAST guidelines for detection of resistance mechanisms and specific resistance of clinical and/or epidemiological importance. EUCAST, version 2.0, July 2017. Available online: https://www.eucast.org/resistance_mechanisms/ (accessed on 9 May 2022).
49. EUCAST. The European Committee on Antimicrobial Susceptibility Testing. Routine and Extended Internal Quality Control for MIC Determination and Disk Diffusion as Recommended by EUCAST, version 6.0–10.0, 2017–2022. Available online: http://www.eucast.org (accessed on 25 November 2022).

antibiotics

MDPI

Article

Staphylococcus aureus and CA-MRSA Carriage among Brazilian Indians Living in Peri-Urban Areas and Remote Communities

Lígia Maria Abraão [1,2,*], Carlos Magno Castelo Branco Fortaleza [1], Carlos Henrique Camargo [3], Thaís Alves Barbosa [1], Eliane Patrícia Lino Pereira-Franchi [1], Danilo Flávio Moraes Riboli [4], Luiza Hubinger [4], Mariana Fávero Bonesso [1], Rodrigo Medeiros de Souza [5] and Maria de Lourdes Ribeiro de Souza da Cunha [1,4,*]

[1] Department of Infectology, Dermatology, Diagnostic Imaging and Radiotherapy, Medical School (FMB) of Sao Paulo State University (UNESP), Botucatu 18618-970, Brazil; carlos.fortaleza@unesp.br (C.M.C.B.F.)

[2] Nursing Research and Care Practices, Hospital Samaritano Higienopolis, São Paulo 01232-010, Brazil

[3] Center of Bacteriology, Adolfo Lutz Institute—IAL, São Paulo 01246-000, Brazil

[4] Department of Chemical and Biological Sciences, Biosciences Institute, UNESP—Universidade Estadual Paulista, Botucatu 18618-691, Brazil

[5] Department of Nursing, Federal University of Acre—UFAC, Cruzeiro do Sul 69920-900, Brazil

* Correspondence: ligia.abraao@americasmed.com.br (L.M.A.); mlrs.cunha@unesp.br (M.d.L.R.d.S.d.C.); Tel.: +55-11-98427-9563 (L.M.A.); +55-14-99798-3735 (M.d.L.R.d.S.d.C.)

Abstract: The emergence of Community-associated methicillin-resistant *Staphylococcus aureus* (CA-MRSA) infections among indigenous populations has been reported. Usually, indigenous communities live in extreme poverty and are at risk of acquiring infections. In Brazil, healthcare inequality is observed in this population. To date, there are no reports of CA-MRSA infections, and no active search for asymptomatic *S. aureus* carriage has been conducted among Brazilian Indians. The aim of this study was to investigate the prevalence of colonization with *S. aureus* and CA-MRSA among Brazilian Indians. We screened 400 Indians (from near urban areas and remote hamlets) for *S. aureus* and CA-MRSA colonization. The isolates were submitted to clonal profiling by pulsed-field gel electrophoresis (PFGE), and selected isolates were submitted to multilocus sequence typing (MLST). Among 931 specimens (nasal and oral) from different indigenous individuals in remote hamlets, *S. aureus* was cultured in 190 (47.6%). Furthermore, CA-MRSA was found in three isolates (0.7%), all SCC*mec* type IV. PFGE analysis identified 21 clusters among the *S. aureus* isolates, and MLST analysis showed a predominance of sequence type 5 among these isolates. Our study revealed a higher prevalence of *S. aureus* carriage among Shanenawa ethnicity individuals (41.1%). Therefore, ethnicity appears to be associated with the prevalence of *S. aureus* in these populations.

Keywords: *Staphylococcus aureus*; CA-MRSA; colonization; brazilian indians; ethnicity; remote communities

1. Introduction

Infections caused by methicillin-resistant *Staphylococcus aureus* (MRSA) are of particular concern because they are harder to treat due to resistance to some antibiotics and because they are no longer limited to healthcare settings [1,2]. On the other hand, globally, strains of methicillin-sensitive *S. aureus* (MSSA) have been associated with a considerable burden of invasive disease, especially among indigenous communities [2–5]. Colonization by *S. aureus* represents a risk factor for the occurrence of autogenous infections and cross-transmission to other individuals [6]. Historically, indigenous populations have been affected by high rates of infectious diseases [2,7,8]. Outbreaks of Community-associated methicillin-resistant *Staphylococcus aureus* (CA-MRSA) were first described among indigenous communities. A remarkable observation was made in Australia in 1980 when a strain of MRSA arose spontaneously in remote Aboriginal communities [9,10]. There is a global trend of considerably higher rates of invasive *S. aureus* disease among indigenous populations [11–14].

According to the most recent Brazilian Census [15], 305 indigenous ethnic groups are found across the Brazilian territory, with a population of 896,917 indigenous people living in the country: 324,834 in urban areas and 572,083 in rural hamlets. Ethnic groups and tribes vary widely in their customs and living conditions, including food, personal hygiene, religious rituals, and housing.

To date, there are no reports of CA-MRSA infections among Brazilian Indigenous, and no active search for asymptomatic *S. aureus* carriage and virulence profile has been conducted. To improve our understanding of *S. aureus* epidemiology among Brazilian Indians, we investigated the contribution of individual, household, and pathogen-related factors associated with *S. aureus* carriage. The objectives of the study were to investigate the prevalence of colonization with overall *S. aureus* and CA-MRSA and virulence factors among Brazilian Indians. We were especially interested in comparing populations living close to urban centers with those from remote areas.

2. Results

A total of 190 *S. aureus* isolates were recovered from the nasal and oral mucosa of 400 individuals (116 from the São Paulo [SP] state and 284 from the Acre [AC] state). The overall prevalence of *S. aureus* colonization was 47.6% (95% confidence interval [CI], 42.6–52.6%) and did not differ among the two study groups (49.5% in AC, 43.1% in SP). Only three subjects (all from AC) carried CA-MRSA, with a prevalence of 0.7% (95% CI: 0.19–2.37). In addition, the CA-MRSA isolates were tested for susceptibility to penicillin, ceftaroline, quinupristin, sulfamethoxazole, clindamycin, erythromycin, and levofloxacin, showing resistance only to penicillin. All CA-MRSA strains harbored SCC*mec* type IV.

Among all *S. aureus* strains, the prevalence of the gene coding for toxic shock syndrome toxin 1 (TSST-1; *tst*) was 6.5%. Among genes encoding enterotoxins, *sec* was the most prevalent (19.9%), followed by *seb* (14.1%) and *sea* (9.4%). The genes for exfoliative toxins A (*eta*) and B (*etb*) were found in 3.6% and 6.8% of the isolates, respectively. Furthermore, 96.3%, 20.4%, and 80.6% of the isolates harbored genes for hemolysins alpha (*hla*), beta (*hlb*), and delta (*hld*), respectively. Biofilm genes (*icaA*, *icaB*, *icaC*, and *icaD*) were detected in 82.2%, 1.0%, 7.8%, and 72.7% of the isolates, respectively. The gene coding for Panton–Valentine leukocidin (PVL; *lukS*-PV) was found in 36 (13.5%) isolates. It is worth noting that all of these isolates were methicillin-susceptible.

In the analysis of risk factors associated with the carriage of *S. aureus*, the univariate Poisson regression model revealed a positive association with age and the number of baths (Table 1). When the factor ethnicity was observed in which the Shanenawa group (the largest group among the indigenous populations studied) was used as a reference, there was a negative association between the Teregua and Kaxinawa ethnicities and the outcome (Table 2). The Shanenawa ethnicity showed a positive association with *S. aureus* carriage when analyzed as a dichotomous variable and was therefore used as the reference in relation to the other ethnicities.

However, in the multivariate analysis, ethnicity was the only independent factor associated with *S. aureus* carriage. The age variable showed a marginally significant *p*-value ($p = 0.08$). Although age and the number of baths did not remain in the multivariate model, they seem to contribute to the outcome studied.

Considering the power of the association of ethnicity with the outcome, univariate analyses were performed comparing the prevalence of virulence factors associated with the ethnic types in order to identify differences in pathogenicity between the *S. aureus* isolates that colonize the indigenous groups studied. From the same perspective, risk factors (habits and customs) were analyzed, and demographic variables (income and the number of household members) were associated with *S. aureus* carriage according to ethnic group. The results show that the Shanenawa ethnicity stands out in relation to the prevalence of the virulence genes, as well as the variables related to habits, customs, and demographics (Tables 2–4).

Table 1. Poisson regression model for the analysis of risk factors associated with *S. aureus*.

Predictors	Univariate Analysis *S. aureus*	Negative	(95% CI)	*p* Value	Multivariate Analysis RR (95% CI)	*p* Value
Demographic Variables						
Women	113 (59.5)	112 (53.6)	1.12 (0.93–1.35)	0.24		
Age, median (quartiles)	21 (11.5–34)	27 (14–43)	...	0.03 *	0.99 (0.98–1.00)	0.08
Ethnicity						
Shanenawa (reference) *	78 (41.1)	57 (27.3)	...	...	1.36 (CI, 1.02–1.82)	0.03 *
Puyanawas I	22 (11.1)	30 (14.4)	0.73 (0.52–1.04)	0.06	0,74 (0.46–1.20)	0.22
Kaxinawa	16 (8.4)	34 (16.3)	0.55 (0.36–0.85)	0.002 *	0.55 (0.32–0.94)	0.03 *
Kopenoti	31 (16.3)	33 (15.8)	0.84 (0.63–1.12)	0.22	0.87 (0.57–1.32)	0.52
Teregua	19 (10.0)	33 (15.8)	0.63 (0.43–0.93)	0.009 *	0.67 (0.40–1.11)	0.11
Ashaninka	4 (2.1)	1 (10.5)	1.34 (0.87–2.20)	0.32	1.32 (0.48–3.62)	0.58
Puyanawas II	21 (11.1)	21 (10.1)	0.87 (0.62–1.21)	0.38	0.91 (0.56–1.38)	0.7
Group (São Paulo x Acre)	50 (26.3)	66 (31.6)	0.89 (0.73–1.08)	0.25		
Income in R$, median (quartiles)	688 (430–800)	700 (422–815)		0.97		
Schooling						
Illiterate (reference)	13 (6.8)	23 (11.0)	...	...		
Incomplete elementary school	77 (40.5)	91 (43.5)	1.27 (0.80–2.002)	0.29		
Continuing						
Univariate Analysis	Multivariate Analysis	Univariate Analysis	Multivariate Analysis	Univariate Analysis	Multivariate Analysis	Univariate Analysis
Complemente elementary school	56 (29.5)	46 (22.0)	1.52 (0.45–2.43)	0.052		
Complete high school	39 (20.5)	41(19.6)	1.35 (0.83–2.20)	0.21		
College degree	5 (2.6)	8 (3.8)	1.07 (0.47–2.40)	1.0		
Brickhouse	60 (31.6)	71 (33.9)	0.95 (0.78–1.16)	0.61		
Sewerage system	85 (44.7)	83 (39.7)	1.10 (0.91–1.51)	0.31		
Number of household members, median (quartiles)	5.5 (4.5–7)	5.0 (3.0–7.5)				
Distance from the health unit, median (quartiles)	2.5 (2.5–5.0)	2.0 (2.0–5.5)		0.52		
Habits and Customs						
Tattoo	18 (9.4)	24 (11.4)	0.90 (0.68–1.20)	0.62		
Collective sports	87 (45.7)	93 (44.5)	1.02 (0.84–1.23)	0.80		
Earrings	45 (32.3)	23 (44.2)	0.69 (0.44–1.10)	0.17		
Skin pigmentation	70 (36.8)	76 (36.3)	1.00 (0.83–1.22)	0.92		
Urucum	55 (29.0)	68 (32.5)	0.92 (0.75–1.12)	0.50		
Jenipapo	67 (35.2)	38 (59.3)	0.85 (0.68–1.08)	0.22		
Number of daily baths, median (quartiles)	3.5 (2.5–4.0)	3.0 (2.0–4.0)	...	0.04 *		
Baths in the river	61 (43.7)	79 (37.8)	0.88 (0.73–1.07)	0.27		
Showers	131 (68.9)	135 (64.5)	1.09 (0.90–1.32)	0.35		
Use of medicinal herbs	33 (17.)	40 (19.1)	0.94 (0.74–1.19)	0.64		
Use of herbal drink for rituals	1 (0.53)	6 (2.87)	0.60 (0.44–0.82)	0.07		
Use of topical medicinal substances	26 (40.6)	38 (59.3)	0.85 (0.68–1.08)	0.22		

Table 1. *Cont.*

Predictors	Univariate Analysis *S. aureus*	Negative	(95% CI)	*p* Value	Multivariate Analysis RR (95% CI)	*p* Value
Drinking	29 (15.2)	32 (15.3)	0.99 (0.77–1.29)	0.98		
Smoking	34 (17.8)	42 (20.1)	0.93 (0.74–1.17)	0.57		
Clinical Variables						
Diabetes	8 (4.2)	11 (5.2)	0.90 (0.60–1.33)	0.62		
Skin infections A	3 (1.58)	2 (0.96)	1.31 (0.44–3.85)	0.57		
Skin infections R	6 (3.16)	8 (3.83)	0.91 (0.57–1.45)	0.71		
Antibiotics	22 (11.5)	19 (9.0)	1.14 (0.81–1.61)	0.41		
Recent outpatient consultations	32 (16.8)	26 (12.4)	1.19 (0.88–1.61)	0.21		
Surgery	17 (8.95)	11 (5.26)	1.35 (0.84–2.17)	0.15		
Hospitalization	27 (14.2)	34 (16.2)	0.92 (0.72–1.18)	0.56		
Pneumonia	1 (0.53)	1 (0.48)	1.04 (0.26–4.20)	0.94		

Data in numbers (%). RR, rate ratio (prevalence ratio); CI confidence interval. * Statistically significant data.

Table 2. Results of the univariate analysis of risk factors associated with *S. aureus* carriage according to ethnicity.

	Shanenawa	Puyanawas I	Puyanawas II	Kaxinawa	Kopenoti	Teregua
Age	21 (11–33)	27 (11–38)	27 (11–49) *	20 (10–34) *	27 (13–42)	31 (13–54) *
Women	71 (52.6%)	24 (47.1%)	29 (69.0%)	28 (56%)	40 (62.5%)	30 (57.7%)
S. aureus	78 (57.8%)	21 (41.2%)	21 (50.0%)	16 (32.0%) *	31 (48.4%)	19 (36.5%)
MRSA	3 (2.2%)	0 (0.0%)	0 (0.0%)	0 (0.0%)	0 (0.0%)	0 (0.0%)
Number of household members, median (quartiles)	6 (4–8)	5 (4–5) *	4 (3–8) *	6 (4–8) *	4 (4–6) *	4 (3–6) *
Number of baths, median (quartiles)	3 (3–4)	3 (3–4)	4 (3–4)	3 (3–4)	2 (1–2) *	2 (2–3) *
Baths in the river	68 (50.4%)	15 (29.4%)	9 (21.4%) *	43 (86.0%) *	0 (0.0%) *	0 (0.0%) *
Tattoo	31 (23%)	3 (5.9%) *	1 (2.4%) *	4 (8.0%) *	0 (0.0%) *	3 (5.8%) *
Skin pigmentation	76 (56.3%)	22 (43.1%)	17 (40.5%)	26 (52.0%)	0 (0.0%) *	0 (0.0%) *
Earrings	1 (0.7%)	0 (0.0%)	0 (0.0%)	0 (0.0%)	1 (1.6%)	2 (3.8%)
Smoking	40 (29.6%)	4 (7.8%) *	7 (16.7%)	10 (20.0%)	7 (10.9%) *	7 (13.5%)
Use of snuff for rituals	1 (0.7%)	1 (2.0)	0 (0.0%)	0 (0.0%)	0 (0.0%)	0 (0.0%)
Use of herbal drink for rituals	1 (0.7%)	6 (11.8%) *	0 (0.0%)	0 (0.0%)	0 (0.0%)	0 (0.0%)
Use of medicinal herbs **	39 (28.9%)	19 (37.3%)	5 (11.9%)	7 (14%)	0 (0.0%) *	1 (1.9%) *
Drinking	39 (28.9%)	5 (9.8%) *	3 (7.1%) *	9 (18.0%)	3 (4.7%) *	1 (1.9%) *
Collective sports	80 (59.3%)	31 (60.8%)	20 (47.6%)	33 (66%)	5 (7.8%) *	10 (19.2%) *

Table 2. *Cont.*

	Shanenawa	Puyanawas I	Puyanawas II	Kaxinawa	Kopenoti	Teregua
Brickhouse	2 (1.5%)	4 (7.8%)	8 (19.0%) *	3 (6.0%)	63 (98.4%) *	51 (98.1%) *
Income in R$, median (quartiles)	632 (334–800) *	600 (400–700) *	670 (490–1000) *	550 (200–684) *	700 (550–750) *	760 (700–1150)

Data in numbers (%).* Statistically significant data. ** Mixture of medicinal herbs typically used by indigenous people for the empirical treatment of diseases.

Table 3. Results of the univariate analysis of risk factors associated with *S. aureus* carriage according to ethnicity.

	Ethnicities—São Paulo & Acre														
	Shanenawa (%)		Puyanawa I (%)		Kaxinawa (%)		Kopenoti (%)		Teregua (%)		Ashaninka (%)		Puyanawas II (%)		*p* Value
Habits and Customs	**Positive**	**Negative**	**Positive**	**Negative**	**Positive**	**Negative**	**Positive**	**Negative**	**Positive**	**Negative**	**Positive**	**Negative**	**Positive**	**Negative**	
Skin pigmentation	76 (52.1)	59 (23.3)	22 (15.1)	29 (11.5)	26 (17.8)	24 (9.5)	-	64 25.6)	-	52 (20.6)	5 (3.4)	-	17 (11.6)	25 (9.9)	<0.01 *
Use of medicinal herbs **	39 (53.4)	96 (29.4)	19 (26.0)	32 (9.8)	7 (9.6)	43 (13.2)	-	64 (19.6)	1 (1.4)	51 (15.6)	2 (2.7)	3 (0.9)	5 (6.8)	37 (11.3)	<0.01 *
Baths in the river	68 (48.6)	67 (25.9)	15 (10.7)	36 (13.9)	43 (30.7)	7 (2.7)	-	64 (24.7)	-	52 (20.1)	5 (3.6)	-	9 (6.4)	33 (12.7)	<0.01 *
Number of baths, median (quartiles)	3.2 (1–4)		3.1 (1–4)		3.2 (1–4)		1.7 (1–4)		2.1 (1–4)		3.0 (2–4)		3.5 (2–4)		
Income in R$, median (quartiles)	696 (50–4000)		781 (70–3550)		505 (60–2000)		810 (134–4000)		1013 (300–2500)		710 (250–1400)		837 (649–4000)		<0.01 *
Household members, median (quartiles)	6.3 (1–20)		4.0 (1–9)		6.0 (2–11)		4.6 (1–9)		3.9 (1–6)		8.0 (8–8)		5.2 (2–11)		<0.01 *

Data in numbers (%). Positive: *S. aureus*. * Statistically significant data. ** Mixture of medicinal herbs typically used by indigenous people for empirical treatment of diseases.

Table 4. Results of the univariate analysis of virulence factors associated with ethnicities.

	Univariate Analysis-Ethnicities—Acre & Sao Paulo State														
	Shanenawa (%)		Puyanawa I (%)		Kaxinawa (%)		Ashaninka (%)		Puyanawas II (%)		Kopenoti-Sp (%)		Teregua-Sp (%)		
Genes	Positive	Negative	Positive	Negative	Positive	Negative	Positive	Negative	Positive	Negative	Positive	Negative	Positive	Negative	*p* Value
S. aureus (*sau*)	78 (41.1)	57 (27.3)	21 (11.1)	30 (14.4)	16 (8.4)	34 (16.3)	4 (2.1)	1 (0.5)	21 (11.1)	21 (10.0)	31 (16.3)	33 (15.8)	19 (10.0)	33 (15.8)	0.01 *
Sea	7 (38.9)	72 (41.6)	1 (5.6)	20 (11.6)	-	16 (9.2)	1 (5.6)	3 (1.7)	1 (5.6)	20 (11.6)	6 (33.3)	25 (14.5)	2 (11.1)	17 (9.8)	0.27
Seb	10 (37.0)	69 (42.1)	1 (3.7)	20 (12.2)	3 (11.1)	13 (7.9)	-	4 (2.4)	2 (7.4)	19 (11.6)	7 (25.9)	24 (14.6)	4 (14.8)	15 (9.1)	0.47
Sec	18 (47.4)	61 (39.9)	5 (13.2)	16 (10.5)	3 (7.9)	13 (8.5)	3 (7.9)	1 (0.7)	4 (10.5)	17 (11.1)	5 (13.2)	26 (17.0)	-	19 (12.4)	0.03 *
Hla	75 (40.8)	4 (57.1)	20 (10.9)	1 (1.3)	15 (8.2)	1 (14.3)	4 (2.2)	-	20 (10.9)	1 (14.3)	31 (16.8)	-	19 (10.3)	-	0.81
Hld	66 (42.9)	13 (35.1)	13 (8.4)	8 (21.6)	11 (7.1)	5 (13.5)	3 (1.9)	1 (2.7)	14 (9.1)	7 (18.9)	29 (18.8)	2 (5.4)	18 (11.7)	1 (2.7)	0.02 *
PVL	14 (38.9)	65 (41.7)	3 (8.3)	18 (11.5)	2 (5.6)	14 (9.0)	1 (2.8)	3 (1.9)	5 (13.9)	16 (10.3)	9 (25.0)	22 (14.1)	2 (5.6)	18 (11.5)	0.62
Eta	5 (71.4)	74 (40.2)	-	21 (11.4)	1 (14.3)	15 (8.2)	-	4 (2.2)	-	21 (11.4)	1 (14.3)	30 (16.3)	-	19 (10.3)	0.62
Etd	5 (38.5)	74 (41.6)	-	21 (11.8)	2 (15.4)	14 (7.9)	-	4 (2.2)	-	21 (11.8)	6 (46.2)	25 (14.0)	-	19 (10.7)	0.03
TSST-1	1 (8.3)	75 (43.6)	-	21 (12.2)	-	15 (8.7)	-	3 (1.7)	-	20 (11.6)	4 (33.3)	26 (15.1)	7 (58.3)	12 (7.0)	<0.01 *
icaA	65 (41.4)	14 (41.2)	20 (12.7)	1 (2.9)	15 (9.6)	1 (2.9)	-	4 (11.8)	20 (12.7)	1 (2.9)	22 (14.0)	9 (26.5)	15 (9.6)	4 (11.8)	<0.01 *
icaD	53 (38.1)	26 (50.0)	17 (12.2)	4 (7.7)	13 (9.4)	3 (5.8)	1 (0.7)	3 (5.8)	20 (14.4)	1 (1.9)	21 (15.1)	10 (19.2)	14 (10.1)	10 (19.2)	004 *

Data in numbers (%). Positive: *S. aureus*. * Statistically significant data.

PFGE typing identified 21 clusters of S. aureus isolates, most of them grouping strains from SP and AC. The dendrogram in Figure 1 shows the electrophoresis typing of the main *S. aureus* clusters identified in indigenous populations from the southeast and northern regions of Brazil. Of these, the following 17 isolates were typed by MLST: ST 5 (4—the most prevalent), ST 8 (2), ST 25 (2), ST 97 (2), ST 188 (2), ST 1 (1), ST 6 (1), ST 15 (1), ST 1635 (1), and SLV 7067 (1).

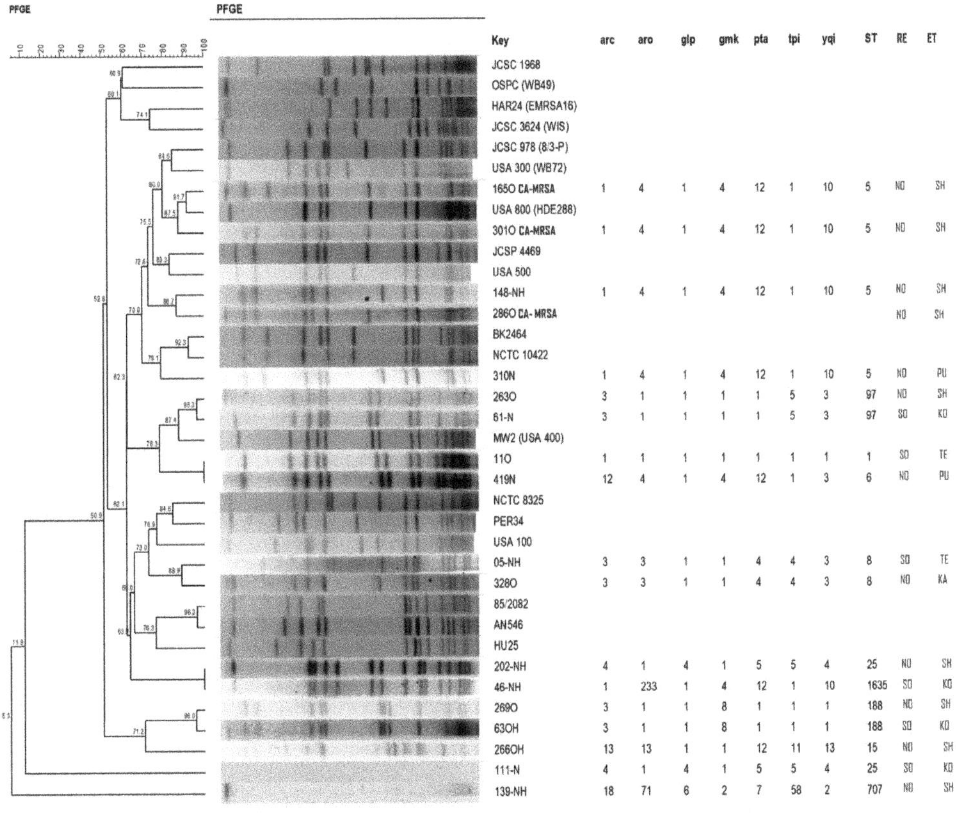

Figure 1. Dendrogram showing pulsed-field gel electrophoresis and multilocus sequence typing of the main S. aureus and CA-MRSA clusters identified in Indian populations from the southeast (SO) and north (NO) regions of Brazil. ST—sequence type; RE—region; ET—ethnicity; SH—Shanenawa; PU—Puyanawa; KO—Kopenoti; TE—Teregua; KA—Kaxinawa.

3. Discussion

In this study, we found that ethnicity was the only predictor associated with *S. aureus* colonization in Brazilian Indians. Furthermore, we identified that income was associated with the prevalence of *S. aureus* carriage among almost all ethnicities. Previous studies also identified a possible association between race, ethnicity, and socioeconomic status, suggesting that these factors seem to contribute to the phenomenon of *S. aureus* colonization [15,16]. Ethnicity is related to the collectivity of individuals, and it is distinguished by their sociocultural specificity, mainly reflected in the language, religion, habits, and living conditions of populations. Considering these facts, it is important to emphasize that most Indian populations live in agglomerations under poor hygiene and sanitation conditions, with large socioeconomic disparities that can contribute to *S. aureus* carriage [17].

The traditional epidemiological factors for *S. aureus* colonization, such as young age, male sex, underlying comorbidities, smoking, and previous hospitalization, were not relevant in the population studied, in agreement with a study investigating an Aboriginal community in Canada [18].

Despite widespread knowledge of the process of *S. aureus* carriage as a predictor of *S. aureus* infections, in Brazil, little is known about the dynamics of colonization and infection with *S. aureus* among indigenous populations. Our study identified a prevalence of *S. aureus* and CA-MRSA carriage of 47.6% and 1.0%, respectively. CA-MRSA strains were restricted to indigenous people belonging to the Amazon region of Brazil, all of them harboring SCC*mec* IV. A study conducted on the Amerindian population of Wayampi in the village of Trois Sauts, an isolated region in the Amazon forest of French Guiana, demonstrated rates of nasal carriage and persistent colonization with *S. aureus* of 57.8% and 26%, respectively. None of the isolates showed resistance to methicillin [19].

Our findings revealed that CA-MRSA was rare and, as also reported in a population-based survey conducted in Brazil, all CA-MRSA harbored SCC*mec* IV [20]. On the other hand, the prevalence of *S. aureus* was higher than that reported for the general population [20]. Antimicrobial susceptibility testing of the MRSA isolates using disks impregnated with penicillin, ceftaroline, quinupristin, sulfamethoxazole, clindamycin, erythromycin, and levofloxacin revealed sensitivity to all antimicrobials, except for penicillin. All isolates were also resistant to penicillin. According to Sader et al. [21], sensitivity rates of CA-MRSA strains are generally higher when compared to hospital-associated MRSA, especially for clindamycin and levofloxacin. The same was observed for ceftaroline, a drug that has recently been introduced on the market as an option for the treatment of infections caused by MRSA.

The results obtained regarding the detection of virulence genes show diversity in the pathogenicity profile of *S. aureus* isolated from indigenous populations, similar to those already identified in non-indigenous populations [22]. Among the most prevalent virulence factors were genes coding for hemolysins *hla* and *hld* and the *icaA* and *icaD* genes involved in biofilm formation. According to Bride et al. [23], these genes are often produced by a large number of *S. aureus* strains. The findings obtained in the present study showed 13.5% of isolates carrying the PVL gene, none of them associated with CA-MRSA. According to Boan et al. [24], infections with PVL-positive *S. aureus* strains disproportionately affect young indigenous people or subjects with fewer healthcare-related risk factors. In a previous study involving a non-indigenous population, only five isolates were found to harbor the gene coding for PVL, corresponding to 2.2% of all isolates [22]. Considering the specific living conditions of the indigenous populations mentioned above, it is possible to infer that such factors may contribute to *S. aureus* carriage and the occurrence of skin infections associated with the PVL gene (*lukS*-PV) [24].

The univariate analyses compared the prevalence of virulence genes associated with ethnicity type and also analyzed the risk factors (habits, customs, and demographic factors) associated with *S. aureus* carriage according to ethnicity; significant results were obtained for the *sec*, *hld*, *tst*, *icaA*, and *icaD* genes. Regarding habits, customs, and demographics, all variables tested were statistically significant: skin pigmentation, number of baths, use of medicinal herbs, baths in the river, monthly income, and number of household members. It is worth noting that individuals of the Shanenawa ethnicity, which was used as a reference and showed a positive association with *S. aureus* when tested as a dichotomous variable, carried the most virulent and resistant *S. aureus* strains. Commonly, this ethnicity more frequently exhibits habits, customs, and demographic factors that may be associated with a higher prevalence of colonization by *S. aureus*.

Regarding PFGE analysis, 21 clusters circulating among the indigenous populations from southeastern and northern Brazil were identified. Of these, five major clusters (1, 4, 6, 10, and 14) contained a larger number of isolates that were more prevalent among the regions studied. Interesting data were observed for these clusters in which isolates from indigenous communities in the southeast formed clusters with isolates identified in the Amazon region. Another interesting finding was that, although not one of the most prevalent, cluster 7 contained sensitive isolates that grouped with one resistant isolate belonging to ST 5. According to Robinson and Enright [25], the dissemination of genotypes occurs not only among individuals but also through the ability to transmit the mobile genetic element SCC*mec* IV through MSSA strains. The remaining CA-MRSA isolates formed clusters with clone USA800. This clone represents a lineage of pandemic MRSA such as CC5 [26].

The sequence type (ST) number 5 was the most frequent. This ST is one of the most prevalent clonal complexes in both hospital and community settings [27,28]. Moreover, the other STs identified in the indigenous populations studied resemble those commonly disseminated in other types of populations [29,30]. ST 5 associates with different types of SCC*mec* (I, II, and IV) and represents the ancestor of the clone described as a Cordobes/Chilean clone and of the MRSA pediatric epidemic clone detected in 1999 [26,31].

4. Materials and Methods

4.1. Study Design, Subjects, and Procedures

A cross-sectional, population-based study was conducted. Individuals of indigenous populations from two different Brazilian states were included. One state was São Paulo, the largest urban center of the country with an area of 1,521,110 km^2 and 11,253,503 inhabitants, and the other state was Acre, located in the remote region of the Amazon forest, which comprises a large area of 8,835,520 km^2 and has 377,057 inhabitants according to IBGE [14].

Our sample size was established by calculating proportions, assuming a level of significance of 5% and accuracy of 5%, according to the number of individuals in each village/hamlet. A total of 400 subjects were included in the study. Of those, 116 lived in a peri-urban village in the city of Bauru, São Paulo State (SP), southeastern Brazil, and 284 lived in small hamlets in Acre State (AC), Brazilian Amazon region. Nasal and oropharyngeal swabs were collected from September to November 2014. Data on demographics (including ethnicity), habits and customs, comorbidities, and clinical variables were collected in interviews with the subjects. Table 5 lists the variables analyzed.

Table 5. Variables included in the analysis.

	Variables Analyzed	
Category	**Description**	**Examples or Additional Information**
Demographic	Gender, age	
	Ethnicity	
	Income in R$	
	Schooling	Illiterate, incomplete elementary school, complete elementary school, complete high school, college degree
	Type of housing	Brickhouse (house built with bricks and cement), houses made of wood/straw or rammed earth
	Sewerage system	
	Median number of household members	
	Distance from the health unit in kilometers	
Habits and customs	Tattoo	
	Collective sports	
	Earrings	
	Skin pigmentation	In general, indigenous peoples have the habit of body painting. In Brazil, dyes are made from natural compounds, such as Urucum and Jenipapo. These dyes remain on the skin for a period of 15 to 20 days.
	Urucum	
	Jenipapo	
	Number of daily baths	Indigenous people living in remote areas have the habit of bathing in the river, and they commonly take many baths throughout the day.
	Baths in the river	
	Use of medicinal herbs	
	Use of herbal drink for rituals	Ayahuasca
	Use of topical medicinal substances	
	Drinking	
	Smoking	Snuff, cigarette

Table 5. *Cont.*

Category	Variables Analyzed Description	Examples or Additional Information
Clinical variables	Diabetes Skin infections A (in the last year) Skin infections R (recent) Antibiotic use Recent outpatient consultations Surgery Hospitalization Pneumonia	

4.2. Specimen Collection, Culture, and Antimicrobial Susceptibility Tests

Nasopharyngeal and oral swabs were collected, transported in Stuart medium, and cultured on a selective medium (Baird-Parker Agar) for up to 48 h. *Staphylococcus aureus* was identified based on colony morphology and standard biochemical tests [32]. Susceptibility to methicillin was tested by disk diffusion using cefoxitin (30 µg) disks according to the recommendations of the Clinical Laboratory Standards Institute [33]. For the MRSA isolates, susceptibility to penicillin, clindamycin, levofloxacin, erythromycin, sulfamethoxazole–trimethoprim, quinupristin–dalfopristin, and ceftaroline was tested by disk diffusion and to oxacillin and vancomycin by the E test (BioMerieux) [32].

4.3. Identification of Virulence Genes

PCR assays for the detection of virulence genes (*sea, seb, sec, hla, hlb, hld, eta, etb, etd, icaA, icaB, icaC,* and *icaD*) were performed following established protocols [34–39]. The primers and references used in this step are listed in Table 6.

Table 6. Primers used for the amplification of toxin and biofilm genes.

Virulence Factor	Gene	Primer	Sequence (5′-3′)	Product	Control	References
Enterotoxin A	*Sea*	SEA-1	TTGGAAACGGTTAAAACGAA	120 bp	ATCC13565	[34,35]
		SEA-2	GAACCTTCCATCAAAAACA			
Enterotoxin B	*seb*	SEB-1	TCGCATCAAACTGACAAACG	478 bp	ATCC 14458	[34,35]
		SEB-2	GACGGTACTCTATAAGTGCC			
Enterotoxin C	*Sec*	SEC-1	GACATAAAAGCTAGGAATTT	257 bp	ATCC 19095	[34,35]
		SEC-2	AAATCGGATTAACATTATCC			
		SEE-2	TAACTTACCGTGGACCCTTC			
Toxic shock syndrome toxin 1	*Tst*	TSST-1	ATGGCAGCATCAGCTTGATA	350 bp	N315	[36]
		TSST-2	TTTCCAATAACCACCCGTTT			
Exfoliative toxin A	*Eta*	ETA-1	CTAGTGCATTTGTTATTCAA	119 bp	N5	[37]
		ETA-2	TGCATTGACACCATAGTACT			
Exfoliative toxin B	*Etb*	ETB-1	ACGGCTATATACATTCAATT	200 bp	ZM	[37]
		ETB-2	TCCATCGATAATATACCTAA			
Exfoliative toxin D	*Etd*	ETD-1	AACTATCATGTATCAAGG	376 bp		[37]
		ETD-2	CAGAATTTCCCGACTCAG			
Hemolysin α	*hla*	HLA-1	CTGATTACTATCCAAGAAATTCGATTG	209 bp	N315	[38]
		HLA-2	CTTTCCAGCCTACTTTTTTATCAGT			
Hemolysin β	*hlb*	HLB-1	GTGCACTTACTGACAATAGTGC	309 bp	RN4420	[38]
		HLB-2	GTTGATGAGTAGCTACCTTCAGT			
Hemolysin δ	*hld*	HLD-1	ATGGCAGCAGATATCATTTC	357 bp	N315	[38]
		HLD-2	CGTGAGCTTGGGAGAGAC			

Table 6. *Cont.*

Virulence Factor	Gene	Primer	Sequence (5′-3′)	Product	Control	References
Biofilm	*ica*A	*ica*A-1	ACA GTC GCT ACG AAA AGA AA	103 bp		[39]
		*ica*A-2	GGA AAT GCC ATA ATG AGA AC			
Biofilm	*ica*B	*ica*B-1	CTG ATC AAG AAT TTA AAT CAC AAA	302 bp		[39]
		*ica*B-2	AAA GTC CCA TAA GCC TGT TT			
Biofilm	*ica*C	*ica*C-1	TAA CTT TAG GCG CAT ATG TTT	400 bp		[39]
		*ica*C-2	TTC CAG TTA GGC TGG TAT TG			
Biofilm	*ica*D	*ica*D-1	ATG GTC AAG CCC AGA CAG AG	198 bp		[39]
		*ica*D-2	CGT GTT TTC AAC ATT TAA TGC AA			

4.4. Molecular Methods

Methicillin resistance was also assessed through the detection of the *mec*A gene by real-time PCR performed in a LightCycler system (Roche) [39]. The staphylococcal cassette chromosome (SCC*mec*) was characterized using the protocol described by Milheiriço et al. [40]. Pulsed-field gel electrophoresis (PFGE) was performed on *Sma*I-digested chromosomal DNA according to the protocol described by McDougal et al. [41]. Band patterns were analyzed with BioNumerics 7.6 (Applied Maths), and a dendrogram was generated using the unweighted pair group method with arithmetic mean (UPGMA). Clusters were defined as any group of more than four isolates with a Dice similarity coefficient $\geq$ 80%, assuming tolerance and optimization of 0.5 and 1.25%, respectively [41].

Representative isolates of the PFGE clusters were submitted to multilocus sequence typing (MLST) [42]. The *arcC*, *aroE*, *glpF*, *gmk*, *pta*, *tpi*, and *yqIL* genes were amplified separately with the specific primers described by Enright et al. [26], and both strands were sequenced. Sequence types (ST) were assigned using the BioNumerics 7.6 software [26].

4.5. Epidemiological Analysis

Data were collected and analyzed using Epi Info for Windows, version 3.5.1 (© Centers for Disease Control and Prevention, Atlanta, GA, USA) and SPSS 20.0 (IBM, Armonk, NY, USA). The base of the study was formed by subjects (indigenous people) with a culture positive for *S. aureus*. Univariate and multivariate Poisson regression models were built. A stepwise forward strategy was used to select variables for the multivariate models, with a *p*-value of 0.05 as a limit for inclusion/removal [42,43].

Figure A1 (Appendix A) shows the workflow of the methodological steps.

4.6. Ethical Issues

This study was approved by the National Committee of Ethics in Research (CONEP/CNS/MS), CAAE: 08428912.3.0000.5411, Approval number 674.368.

5. Conclusions

In conclusion, ethnicity appears to be associated with a higher prevalence of *S. aureus* and virulence in special populations, even though the prevalence of CA-MRSA was low. These results might be related to specific habits and customs since poor housing conditions, hygiene, and sanitation are features present in most ethnical groups and can influence the carriage and dissemination of *S. aureus* among populations. It is, therefore, extremely important that these factors be considered for the development and implementation of strategies designed to control the spread of microorganisms among different human populations, especially considering the health inequality of indigenous populations in Brazil.

Author Contributions: Conceptualization, L.M.A., M.d.L.R.d.S.d.C. and C.M.C.B.F.; methodology, L.M.A., R.M.d.S., T.A.B., C.H.C., M.F.B., L.H. and E.P.L.P.-F.; software, D.F.M.R. and C.H.C.; formal analysis, C.M.C.B.F.; writing—original draft preparation, L.M.A.; writing—review and editing, L.M.A., M.d.L.R.d.S.d.C., C.H.C. and C.M.C.B.F.; supervision, M.d.L.R.d.S.d.C. and C.M.C.B.F.; project administration, L.M.A. All authors have read and agreed to the published version of the manuscript.

Funding: Coordination for the Improvement of Higher Education Personnel (CAPES, number: 110938-3) and National Council for Scientific and Technological Development (CNPq—Grant 303603/2020-8).

Institutional Review Board Statement: This study was conducted in accordance with the Declaration of Helsinki, and approved by the National Committee of Ethics in Research (CONEP/CNS/MS), protocol code 08428912.3.0000.5411, approval number: 674.368, 06/09/2014.

Informed Consent Statement: Informed consent was obtained from all subjects involved in the study.

Data Availability Statement: The data presented in this study are original and have not been published in scientific journals. The only document that contains these data is the doctoral thesis of Lígia Maria Abraão, openly available in [Institutional Repository of UNESP] at [https://repositorio.unesp.br/handle/11449/151310?locale-attribute=en] (accessed on 1 March 2023).

Conflicts of Interest: All authors declare no conflict of interest.

Appendix A

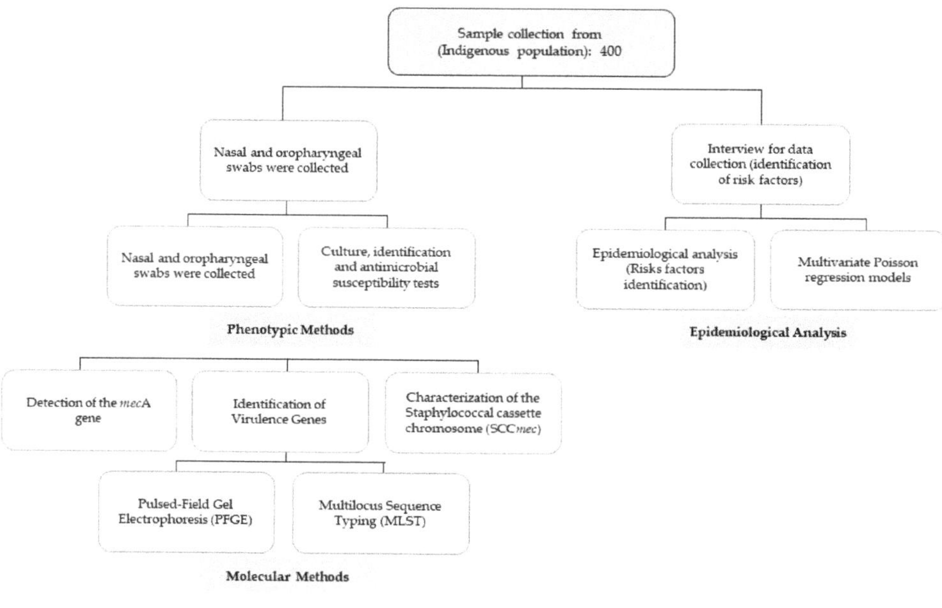

Figure A1. Workflow of the methodological steps.

References

1. David, M.Z.; Daum, R.S. Community-associated methicillin-resistant *Staphylococcus aureus*: Epidemiology and clinical consequences of an emerging epidemic. *Clin. Microbiol. Rev.* **2010**, *23*, 616–687. [CrossRef]
2. Sutcliffe, C.G.; Grant, L.R. High Burden of *Staphylococcus aureus* Among Native American Individuals on the White Mountain Apache Tribal Lands. *Open Forum Infect. Dis.* **2020**, *7*, ofaa061. [CrossRef]
3. Kanjilal, S.; Sater, M.R.A. Trends in antibiotic susceptibility in *Staphylococcus aureus* in Boston, Massachusetts, from 2000 to 2014. *J. Clin. Microbiol.* **2018**, *56*, e01160-17. [CrossRef]
4. Sutcliffe, C.G.; Grant, L.R. The burden of *Staphylococcus aureus* among Native Americans on the Navajo Nation. *PLoS ONE* **2019**, *14*, e0213207. [CrossRef] [PubMed]

5. Cella, C.; Sutcliffe, C.G. Carriage prevalence and genomic epidemiology of *Staphylococcus aureus* among Native American children and adults in the Southwestern USA. *Microb. Genom.* **2022**, *8*, mgen000806. [CrossRef] [PubMed]
6. Mehraj, J.; Witte, W. Epidemiology of *Staphylococcus aureus* Nasal Carriage Patterns in the Community. *Curr. Top. Microbiol. Immunol.* **2016**, *398*, 55–87. [PubMed]
7. Butler, J.C.; Crengle, S. Emerging infectious diseases among indigenous peoples. *Emerg. Infect. Dis.* **2001**, *7*, 554–555. [CrossRef] [PubMed]
8. Landen, M.G.; McCumber, B.J. Asam ED, Egeland GM. Outbreak of boils in an Alaskan village: A case-control study. *West. J. Med.* **2000**, *172*, 235–239. [CrossRef]
9. Groom, A.V.; Wolsey, D.H. Community-acquired methicillin-resistant *Staphylococcus aureus* in a rural American Indian community. *JAMA* **2001**, *286*, 1201–1205. [CrossRef] [PubMed]
10. Muileboom, J.; Hamilton, M. Community-associated methicillin-resistant *Staphylococcus aureus* in northwest Ontario: A five-year report of incidence and antibiotic resistance. *Can. J. Infect. Dis. Med. Microbiol.* **2013**, *24*, e42–e44. [CrossRef] [PubMed]
11. Abelson, W.H.; Banerji, A. Community-associated methicillin-resistant *Staphylococcus aureus* in indigenous communities in Canada. *Paediatr. Child. Health* **2012**, *17*, 395–398.
12. Ng, J.W.S.; Holt, D.C. Phylogenetically distinct *Staphylococcus aureus* lineage prevalent among indigenous communities in northern Australia. *J. Clin. Microbiol.* **2009**, *47*, 2295–2300. [CrossRef] [PubMed]
13. Tong, S.Y.C.; Varrone, L. Progressive increase in community-associated methicillin-resistant *Staphylococcus aureus* in indigenous populations in northern Australia from 1993 to 2012. *Epidemiol. Infect.* **2015**, *143*, 1519–1523. [CrossRef]
14. IBGE. Instituto Brasileiro de Geografia e Estatística [Internet]. Brazil: Censo Polulações Indígenas. Available online: https://www.gov.br/funai/pt-br/assuntos/noticias/2022-02/ultimo-censo-do-ibge-registrou-quase-900-mil-indigenas-no-pais-dados-serao-atualizados-em-2022#:~:text=%C3%9Altimo%20censo%20do%20IBGE%20regi-trou,Funda%C3%A7%C3%A3o%20Nacional%20dos%20Povos%20Ind%C3%ADgenas (accessed on 12 February 2023).
15. Tong, S.Y.; McDonald, M.I. Global implications of the emergence of community-associated methicillin-resistant *Staphylococcus aureus* in Indigenous populations. *Clin. Infect. Dis.* **2008**, *46*, 1871–1878. [CrossRef]
16. Wertheim, H.F.; Melles, D.C. The role of nasal carriage in *Staphylococcus aureus* infections. *Lancet Infect. Dis.* **2005**, *12*, 751–762. [CrossRef] [PubMed]
17. Verhagen, L.M.; Hermsen, M. Nasopharyngeal carriage of respiratory pathogens in Warao Amerindians: Significant relationship with stunting. *Trop. Med. Int. Health* **2017**, *22*, 407–414. [CrossRef] [PubMed]
18. Daley, P.; Bajgai, J. A cross sectional study of animal and human colonization with methicillin-resistant *Staphylococcus aureus* (MRSA) in an Aboriginal community. *BMC Public. Health* **2016**, *16*, 1–7. [CrossRef]
19. Ruimy, R.; Angebault, C.C. Are host genetics the predominant determinant of persistent nasal *Staphylococcus aureus* carriage in humans? *J. Infect. Dis.* **2010**, *202*, 924–934. [CrossRef]
20. Pires, F.V.; Da Cunha, M.D.L.R.D.S. Nasal carriage of *Staphylococcus aureus* in Botucatu, Brazil: A population-based survey. *PLoS ONE* **2014**, *9*, e92537. [CrossRef]
21. Sader, H.S.; Gales, A.C. Pathogen frequency and resistance patterns in Brazilian hospitals: Summary of results from three years of the SENTRY Antimicrobial Surveillance Program. *Braz. J. Infect. Dis.* **2001**, *5*, 200–214. [CrossRef]
22. Abraão, L.M. Detection of Virulence Genes and Identification of the Clonal Profile of Staphylococcus aureus Isolates Colonizing the Nasopharynx Obtained in a Popular Base Study. Master's Degree. Paulista State University "Júlio de Mesquita Filho" (UNESP), Botucatu, São Paulo State, Brazil, February 2013. Available online: https://repositorio.unesp.br/handle/11449/110458?show=full (accessed on 20 February 2023).
23. Bride, L.L.; Pereira, M.F. Differences in resistance profiles and virulence genes among methicillin-resistant and methicillin-susceptible *Staphylococcus aureus* of different lineages at a public tertiary hospital. *Rev. Soc. Bras. Med. Trop.* **2019**, *52*, e20190095. [CrossRef]
24. Boan, P.; Tan, H. Epidemiological, clinical, outcome and antibiotic susceptibility differences between PVL positive and PVL negative *Staphylococcus aureus* infections in Western Australia: A case control study. *BMC Infect. Dis.* **2015**, *15*, 10. [CrossRef] [PubMed]
25. Robinson, D.A.; Enright, M.C. Evolutionary models of the emergence of methicillin-resistant *Staphylococcus aureus*. *Antimicrob. Agents Chemother.* **2003**, *47*, 3926–3934. [CrossRef] [PubMed]
26. Enright, M.C.; Day, N.P.J. Multilocus sequence typing for characterization of methicillin-resistant and methicillin-susceptible clones of *Staphylococcus aureus*. *J. Clin. Microbiol.* **2000**, *38*, 1008–1015. [CrossRef] [PubMed]
27. Shettigar, K.; Murali, T.S. Virulence factors and clonal diversity of *Staphylococcus aureus* in colonization and wound infection with emphasis on diabetic foot infection. *Eur. J. Clin. Microbiol. Infect. Dis.* **2020**, *39*, 2235–2246. [CrossRef]
28. McGuinness, S.L.; Holt, D.C. Clinical and molecular epidemiology of an emerging Panton Valentine leukocidin-positive ST5 methicillin-resistant *Staphylococcus aureus* clone in northern Australia. *mSphere* **2021**, *6*, e00651-20. [CrossRef] [PubMed]
29. Jian, Y.; Zhao, L. Increasing Prevalence of Hypervirulent ST5 Methicillin Susceptible *Staphylococcus aureus* Subtype Poses a Serious Clinical Threat. *Emerg. Microbes Infect.* **2020**, *10*, 109–122. [CrossRef] [PubMed]
30. Witzel, C.; Fortaleza, C.M.C.B. Nasopharyngeal carriage of *Staphylococcus aureus* among imprisoned males from Brazil without exposure to healthcare: Risk factors and molecular characterization. *Ann. Clin. Microbiol. Antimicrob.* **2014**, *13*, 25. [CrossRef] [PubMed]

31. Sola, C.; Paganini, H. Spread of epidemic MRSA-ST5-IV clone encoding PVL as a major cause of community onset staphylococcal infections in Argentinean children. *PLoS ONE* **2012**, *7*, e30487. [CrossRef] [PubMed]
32. Konemman, E.V.; Allen, S.D. Introdução à microbiologia médica. In *Diagnóstico Microbiológico: Texto e Atlas Colorido*, 5th ed.; Medsi: Rio de Janeiro, Brazil, 2001; pp. 200–210.
33. Clinical and Laboratory Standards Institute. *Performance Standards for Antimicrobial Disk Susceptibility Tests*, 31st ed.; CLSI Supplement M100; Clinical and Laboratory Standards Institute: Wayne, PE, USA, 2021.
34. Johnson, W.M.; Tyler, S.D. Detection of genes for enterotoxins, exfoliative toxins, and toxic shock syndrome toxin 1 in *Staphylococcus aureus* by the polymerase chain reaction. *J. Clin. Microbiol.* **1991**, *29*, 426–430. [CrossRef]
35. Cunha, M.D.L.R.S.; Calsolari, R.O. Detection of enterotoxin and toxic shock syndrome toxin 1 genes in *Staphylococcus*, with emphasis on coagulase-negative staphylococci. *Microbiol. Immunol.* **2007**, *51*, 381–390. [CrossRef] [PubMed]
36. Marconi, C.; Cunha, M.L.R.S. Standardization of the PCR technique for the detection of delta toxin in *Staphylococcus* spp. *J. Venom. Anim. Toxins Incl. Trop. Dis.* **2005**, *11*, 117–128. [CrossRef]
37. Koning, S.; Van, B.A. Severity of nonbullous *Staphylococcus aureus* impetigo in children is associated with strains harboring genetic markers for exfoliative toxin B, Panton-Valentine leukocidin, and the multidrug resistance plasmid pSK41. *J. Clin. Microbiol.* **2003**, *41*, 3017–3021. [CrossRef] [PubMed]
38. Arciola, C.R.; Gamberini, S. A multiplex PCR method for the detection of all five individual genes of ica locus in Staphylococcus epidermidis. A survey on 400 clinical isolates from prosthesis-associated infections. *J. Biomed. Mater. Res. A* **2005**, *75*, 408–413. [CrossRef] [PubMed]
39. Fang, H.; Hedin, G. Rapid Screening and Identification of Methicillin-Resistant *Staphylococcus aureus* from Clinical Samples by Selective-Broth and Real-Time PCR Assay. *J. Clin. Microbiol.* **2003**, *41*, 2894–2899. [CrossRef]
40. Milheirico, C.; Oliveira, D.C. Update to the multiplex PCR strategy for assignment of mec element types in *Staphylococcus aureus*. *Antimicrob. Agents Chemother.* **2007**, *51*, 4537. [CrossRef]
41. McDougal, L.K.; Steward, C.D. Pulsed-field gel electrophoresis typing of oxacillin-resistant *Staphylococcus aureus* isolates from the United States: Establishing a National Database. *J. Clin. Microbiol.* **2003**, *41*, 5113–5120. [CrossRef]
42. Coutinho, L.M.S.; Scazufca, M. Methods for estimating prevalence ratios in cross-sectional studies. *Rev. Saude Publica* **2008**, *42*, 992–998. [CrossRef] [PubMed]
43. Barros, A.J.D.; Hirakata, V.N. Alternatives for logistic regression in cross-sectional studies: An empirical comparison of models that directly estimate the prevalence ratio. *BMC Med. Res. Methodol.* **2003**, *21*, 21. [CrossRef]

antibiotics

MDPI

Article

Multi-Drug Resistant *Staphylococcus aureus* Carriage in Abattoir Workers in Busia, Kenya

Benear Apollo Obanda [1,2,3], Cheryl L. Gibbons [4], Eric M. Fèvre [5,6,*], Lilly Bebora [1], George Gitao [1], William Ogara [7], Shu-Hua Wang [2,8], Wondwossen Gebreyes [2,9], Ronald Ngetich [3], Beth Blane [10], Francesc Coll [11], Ewan M. Harrison [10,12,13], Samuel Kariuki [3], Sharon J. Peacock [10] and Elizabeth A. J. Cook [6,*]

1 Department of Veterinary Pathology, Microbiology and Parasitology, University of Nairobi, Nairobi P.O. Box 29053-00625, Kenya
2 Global One Health Initiative, The Ohio State University, Columbus, OH 43210, USA
3 Centre for Microbiology Research Nairobi, Kenya Medical Research Institute, Nairobi P.O. Box 54840-00200, Kenya
4 Public Health Scotland, Glasgow G2 6QE, UK
5 Institute of Infection, Veterinary & Ecological Sciences, Leahurst Campus, University of Liverpool, Chester High Road, Neston CH64 7TE, UK
6 International Livestock Research Institute, Nairobi P.O. Box 30709-00100, Kenya
7 Department of Public Health Pharmacology and Toxicology, University of Nairobi, Nairobi P.O. Box 29053-00625, Kenya
8 Division of Infectious Disease, Department of Internal Medicine, The Ohio State University, Columbus, OH 43210, USA
9 Department of Veterinary Preventive Medicine, College of Veterinary Medicine, The Ohio State University, Columbus, OH 43210, USA
10 Department of Medicine, University of Cambridge, Cambridge CB2 0QQ, UK
11 London School of Hygiene and Tropical Medicine, London WC1E 7HT, UK
12 Wellcome Sanger Institute, Hinxton CB10 1SA, UK
13 Department of Public Health and Primary Care, University of Cambridge, Cambridge CB1 8RN, UK
* Correspondence: eric.fevre@liverpool.ac.uk (E.M.F.); e.cook@cgiar.org (E.A.J.C.)

Abstract: Abattoir workers have been identified as high-risk for livestock-associated *Staphylococcus aureus* carriage. This study investigated *S. aureus* carriage in abattoir workers in Western Kenya. Nasal swabs were collected once from participants between February-November 2012. *S. aureus* was isolated using bacterial culture and antibiotic susceptibility testing performed using the VITEK 2 instrument and disc diffusion methods. Isolates underwent whole genome sequencing and Multi Locus Sequence Types were derived from these data. *S. aureus* ($n = 126$) was isolated from 118/737 (16.0%) participants. Carriage was higher in HIV-positive (24/89, 27.0%) than HIV–negative participants (94/648, 14.5%; $p = 0.003$). There were 23 sequence types (STs) identified, and half of the isolates were ST152 (34.1%) or ST8 (15.1%). Many isolates carried the Panton-Valentine leucocidin toxin gene (42.9%). Only three isolates were methicillin resistant *S. aureus* (MRSA) (3/126, 2.4%) and the prevalence of MRSA carriage was 0.4% (3/737). All MRSA were ST88. Isolates from HIV-positive participants (37.0%) were more frequently resistant to sulfamethoxazole/trimethoprim compared to isolates from HIV-negative participants (6.1%; $p < 0.001$). Similarly, trimethoprim resistance genes were more frequently detected in isolates from HIV-positive (81.5%) compared to HIV-negative participants (60.6%; $p = 0.044$). *S. aureus* in abattoir workers were representative of major sequence types in Africa, with a high proportion being toxigenic isolates. HIV-positive individuals were more frequently colonized by antimicrobial resistant *S. aureus* which may be explained by prophylactic antimicrobial use.

Keywords: *S. aureus*; MSSA; MRSA; abattoir; slaughterhouse; Kenya; HIV; AMR; antimicrobial resistance

1. Introduction

Staphylococcus aureus is a common commensal of the skin, thought to persistently colonize approximately one third of the human population [1]. Nasal carriage of *S. aureus* is a recognized risk factor for skin and soft tissue infections (SSTI) in the clinical setting [2,3]. *S. aureus* may also cause food poisoning and more serious conditions such as pneumonia, endocarditis, osteomyelitis, sepsis, and toxic shock syndrome [4]. HIV-positive individuals are more likely to be colonized by *S. aureus*, which accounts for significant morbidity in this group compared to the general population [5].

The sub-Saharan region is recognized as the world's epicenter of the HIV/AIDS epidemic. The prevalence of HIV in Kenya is 5% [6]. The Kenyan Ministry of Health recommends the use of sulfamethoxazole/trimethoprim for the management of opportunistic infections in all HIV positive patients regardless of immunological status [7]. The prophylactic use of sulfamethoxazole/trimethoprim in HIV-positive individuals results in significant protection from a range of pathogens including *Toxoplasma gondii*, *Salmonella* sp., *Haemophilus* sp., *Staphylococcus* sp., and *Pneumocystis jiroveci* [8]. However, prophylactic use of sulfamethoxazole/trimethoprim in HIV-positive individuals in the sub-Saharan region has led to the emergence of antibiotic resistant and multidrug resistant *S. aureus* strains [9,10].

Antimicrobial resistance (AMR) poses a threat to life since infections caused by multidrug resistant organisms have fewer treatment options available [11]. This is particularly important for the HIV-positive population. Injudicious use of antibiotics in human medicine, coupled with extensive antibiotic use in livestock production for both therapeutic and non-therapeutic reasons has led to the development of antibiotic resistant bacteria in people and animals [12,13]. Multi-drug resistant methicillin sensitive *S. aureus* (MSSA) and methicillin resistant *S. aureus* (MRSA) have been detected in animals and meat products [14]. There has also been documented transmission to livestock keepers and abattoir workers [15,16]. This implies that, abattoir workers' nares can be colonized by *S. aureus* from contaminated meat, transforming them into carriers or reservoirs of *S. aureus*. Carriers can transmit the bacteria from their noses to other body parts, to the general population, or contaminate foods and food surfaces during handling [17]. These transmission routes have been reported in several European countries [18,19].

Multi-locus sequence typing is conducted on *S. aureus* to understand the molecular epidemiology of the isolates including the evolution, source attribution and transmission through the sequencing of seven housekeeping genes [20]. Clonal complexes (CC) describe *S. aureus* lineages by grouping sequence types (STs) where at least 5/7 alleles are identical between STs in the group [21]. The dominant STs vary between countries and within countries depending on the source. The dominant MSSA STs in Africa are ST5, ST8, ST15, ST30, ST121, ST152 and the dominant MRSA STs are ST5, ST8, ST80, ST88, ST239/ST241 [22]. There is limited information of the predominant sequence types in Kenya but there are increased reports of ST5, ST8, ST22, with the predominant MRSA ST being ST239/241 [23–28].

Isolates of *S. aureus* may carry genes for virulence factors such as Panton-Valentine leukocidin (PVL), and the toxic shock syndrome toxin (TSST-1) [29–31]. PVL is a virulence factor which is associated with SSTI and has a debatable role in causing necrotizing pneumonia [32–35] whereas TSST-1 results in toxic shock syndrome leading to lethal hypotension [29]. In sub-Saharan Africa *S. aureus* isolates more frequently carry the *pvl* gene with the median prevalence of *pvl*-positive MRSA being 33% (range from 0 to 77%; $n = 15$), compared to Europe where less than 5% of *S. aureus* isolates carry the *pvl* gene [23,36,37]. There is very little information about the prevalence of *tsst-1* gene carriage in Africa with one study in Nigeria reporting carriage in human isolates to be 16% [38].

Here, we report on a study of MSSA/MRSA nasal carriage of abattoir workers in rural abattoirs in Busia County, western Kenya. This study aimed to establish the prevalence of MSSA and MRSA colonization and describe genetic characteristics of isolates obtained from abattoir workers in order to understand the epidemiology of *S. aureus* in this population of workers exposed to livestock. This was done by investigating the prevalence of *pvl* and *tsst-1* genes, antimicrobial susceptibility and diversity of STs. Due to the high proportion of HIV-positive individuals in this population we also endeavored to use this dataset to understand the effect of prophylactic use of sulfamethoxazole/trimethoprim in HIV-positive individuals on the emergence of MSSA/MRSA antibiotic resistance and associated virulence by comparing HIV-positive and HIV-negative workers. Genotypic characterization of virulent strains and their antibiotic resistance profiles will contribute to understanding the potential sources and transmission routes of *S. aureus* in this setting. This information will be valuable to Kenya's National Policy for the prevention and containment of AMR [39].

2. Results

2.1. Description of Study Population

A total of 737/738 abattoir workers, recruited between February and November 2012, consented to a blood sample and a single nasal swab which was cultured for the presence of *S. aureus*. One participant declined to provide a blood sample and was excluded.

The majority of participants were men 711/737 (96.5%) and the mean age was 39 (range 18–82 years). The number of participants who tested positive for HIV was 89/737 (12.1%, 95%CI 9.9–14.7%). Additionally, 127/737 (17.2%) of participants had taken antibiotics in the previous month.

2.2. Prevalence of MRSA and MSSA among HIV-Positive and HIV-Negative Participants

S. aureus was isolated from 118/737 (16.0%; 95%CI 13.6–18.8%) participants. From 118 positive samples, 126 isolates were cultured in total since four participants had two separate strains and a further two participants had three strains identified from the same sample. Three isolates were MRSA and 123 isolates were MSSA, giving a prevalence of MRSA carriage of 0.4% (95%CI 0.1–1.2%), and MSSA carriage of 15.6 % (95%CI 13.2–18.5%), respectively (Table 1). There were no known relationships between the three MRSA carriers, and individuals worked at different abattoirs.

Table 1. Prevalence of MSSA and MRSA isolated from Abattoir workers in Busia County.

HIV-Status	Number of *S. aureus* Isolates (Number of MRSA)	Number of Workers Who Yielded *Staph. aureus* (%, 95% Confidence Interval)	Number of Workers Carrying MRSA Isolates (%, 95%CI)	Number of Workers Carrying MSSA Isolates (%, 95%CI)
HIV-positive (n = 89)	27 (1)	24 (27.0%, 95%CI 18.9–37.1)	1 (1.1%, 95%CI 0.3–6.0)	23 (25.8%, 95%CI 18.0–26.0)
HIV-negative (n = 648)	99 (2)	94 (14.5%, 95%CI 11.9–17.4)	2 (0.3%, 95%CI 0.1–1.1)	92 (14.2%, 95%CI 11.7–17.1)
Total abattoir workers (n = 737)	126 (3)	118 (16.0%, 95%CI 13.5–29.0)	3 (0.4%, 95%CI 0.1–1.2)	115 (15.6%, 95%CI 13.1–18.3)

Of the HIV-positive workers, 24/89 were positive for *S. aureus* (27.0% (95%CI 19.1–36.7%). In contrast, 94/648 HIV-negative workers were positive for *S. aureus* (14.5%, 95%CI 12.0–17.4%) (Chi^2 = 9.081, df = 1, p = 0.003). There were 27 *S. aureus* isolates cultured from HIV-positive workers (26 MSSA and 1 MRSA) and 99 *S. aureus* isolates from HIV-negative individuals (97 MSSA and 2 MRSA). There was no difference in detection of MRSA in the two groups (HIV-negative 2/99, 2.0% versus HIV-positive 1/27, 3.7%; Chi^2 = 0.263, df = 1, p = 0.608). There was no significant difference between the proportion of HIV-positive workers (17/89, 19.1%) and HIV-negative workers (110/647, 17.0%) who had recently taken antibiotics (Chi^2 = 0.241, df = 1, p = 0.623).

2.3. Genetic Diversity of MSSA and MRSA STs in HIV-Positive and HIV-Negative Participants

Multi-locus sequence typing from the whole genome sequencing of the 126 *S. aureus* isolates identified eleven clonal complexes, consisting of CC1, CC5, CC8, CC15, CC22, CC25, CC30, CC72, CC80, and CC88 (Figure 1). The largest cluster of isolates was CC152. Two ST types accounted for approximately half of all isolates with ST152 (43/126, 34.1%), and ST8 (19/126, 15.1%,) most frequently identified, followed by ST72 (9/126, 7.1%), ST80 (7/126, 5.6%) and ST22 (5/126, 4%). The three MRSA isolates were all ST88.

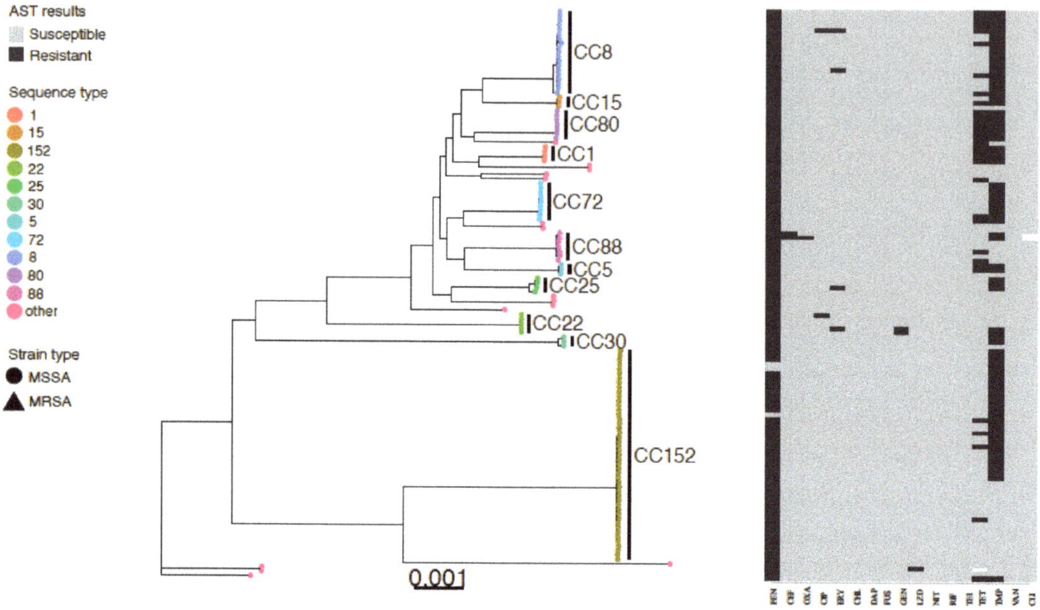

Figure 1. Core genome phylogenetic tree and antibiogram of MSSA and MRSA isolates colonizing abattoir workers in western Kenya. Predominant ST types are differentiated by colour, MRSA isolates are indicated by a triangle symbol and MSSA by circles. Phenotypic antimicrobial resistance is indicated by dark grey bars (resistant), white bars (intermediate), and light grey (susceptible). Antimicrobials: PEN—benzylpenicillin, CEF—cefoxitin, OXA—oxacillin, CIP—ciprofloxacin, ERY—erythromycin, CHL—chloramphenicol, DAP—daptomycin, FUS—fusidic acid, GEN—gentamicin, LZD- linezolid, NIT—nitrofurantoin, RIF—rifampicin, TEI—teicoplanin, TET—tetracycline, TMP—trimethoprim, VAN—vancomycin, CLI—clindamycin.

HIV-positive participants carried 8 different STs and HIV-negative participants carried 23 different STs, indicating roughly equivalent genetic diversity in the two groups. There was no difference in the carriage of ST152 in HIV-negative (35/99, 35.4%) versus HIV-positive participants (8/27, 29.6%; Chi^2 = 0.315, df = 1, p = 0.575). ST8 was isolated at a higher proportion from HIV-positive (11/27, 40.7%) than HIV-negative participants (8.1%, 8/99) (Chi^2 = 17.460, df = 1, $p < 0.001$). All ST72 were recovered from HIV-negative participants (Supplementary Table S1).

2.4. Prevalence of PVL Gene and Toxic Shock Syndrome Toxin-1 (TSST-1) Gene Carriage

Almost half of isolates (54/126, 42.9%) were *pvl*-positive. There was no difference in prevalence of *pvl* gene carriage between isolates from HIV-positive workers (10/27, 37.0%) and isolates from HIV-negative participants (44/99, 44.4%; Chi^2 = 0.471, df = 1, p = 0.493). The majority of *pvl*-positive isolates were ST152 (39/54, 72.2%). Other STs, with *pvl* gene carriage were ST1633 (4/54, 7.4%), ST30 (3/53, 5.6%), ST88 (2/54, 3.7%), ST80 (2/54, 3.7%), ST2430 (1/54, 1.9%), ST22 (1/54, 1.9%), and ST5 (1/54, 1.9%). The *tsst-1* gene was identified in 15/126 isolates (11.9%), the majority of which were ST 72 (9/15, 60%). The remainder were ST22 (3/15, 20%), ST707 (2/15, 13.3%) and ST8 (1/15, 6.7%). The majority of *tsst-1* positive isolates (n = 14) were detected in HIV-negative participants. The three MRSA isolates were negative for both genes.

2.5. Prevalence of Phenotypic Antibiotic Resistant S. aureus Carriage in Participants

Antibiotic susceptibility testing of the 126 *S. aureus* isolates using the VITEK 2 instrument demonstrated that all isolates were susceptible to chloramphenicol, daptomycin, fusidic acid, mupirocin, nitrofurantoin, rifampicin, teicoplanin, tigecycline, vancomycin, and clindamycin. Resistance was very low to cefoxitin (2/126, 1.6%), ciprofloxacin (2/126, 1.6%), erythromycin (4/126, 3.2%), gentamicin (2/126, 1.6 %), linezolid (1/126, 0.8 %), oxacillin (1/126, 0.8%), and inducible resistance to clindamycin (4/126, 3.2%). Higher levels of resistance were detected to penicillin-G (123/126, 97.6%); trimethoprim (81/126, 64.3%), tetracycline (33/126, 26.2%) by VITEK 2, and sulfamethoxazole/trimethoprim by disc diffusion (16/126, 12.7%) (Table 2).

Table 2. Prevalence of antibiotic resistant *Staph. aureus* carriage among HIV-positive and HIV-negative abattoir workers in Busia County.

	Total Number of Isolates n = 126 (%)	Isolates from HIV-Positive Workers n = 27 (%)	Isolates from HIV-Negative Workers n = 99 (%)	Chi^2 Test
Sulfamethoxazole/ trimehoprim resistance	16 (12.7)	10 (37.0)	6 (6.1)	Chi^2 = 18.098, df = 1, p <0.001
Penicillin	123 (97.6)	26 (100)	96 (97.0)	NA
Trimethoprim	81 (64.3)	21 (77.8)	60 (60.6)	Chi^2 = 2.712, df = 1, p = 0.100
Cefoxitin	2 (1.6%)	1 (3.7)	2 (2.0)	Chi^2 = 0.263, df = 1, p = 0.608
Tetracycline	33 (26.2)	10 (37.0)	23 (23.2)	Chi^2 = 2.075, df = 1, p = 0.150
Erythromycin	4 (3.2)	2 (7.4)	2 (2.0)	Chi^2 = 2.007, df = 1, p = 0.157
Inducible resistance to clindamycin	4 (3.2)	2 (7.4)	2 (2.0)	Chi^2 = 2.007, df = 1, p = 0.157
Gentamicin	2 (1.6)	0	2 (2.0)	NA
Ciprofloxacin	2 (1.6)	2 (7.4)	0	NA
Oxacillin	1 (0.8)	0	1 (1.0)	NA
Linezolid	1 (0.8)	0	1 (1.0)	NA
Panton Valentine Leukocidin gene	54 (42.9)	10 (37.0)	44 (44.4)	Chi^2 = 0.471, df = 1, p = 0.493
Toxic shock syndrome toxin-1 gene	15 (11.9)	1 (3.7)	14 (14.1)	Chi^2 = 2.176, df = 1, p = 0.140
Multidrug-resistant	34 (27.0)	9 (33.3)	25 (25.3)	Chi^2 =0.683, df = 1, p = 0.409
Trimethoprim-Penicillin-Tetracycline MDR	28 (22.2)	8 (29.6)	20 (20.2)	Chi^2 = 1.076, df = 1, p = 0.230

Resistance to trimethoprim was not significantly different between isolates from HIV-positive (21/27, 77.8%) and HIV negative (60/90, 60.6%) participants (Chi^2 = 2.712, df = 1, p = 0.100). In contrast, resistance to sulfamethoxazole/trimethoprim by disc diffusion was more common in HIV-positive participants (10/27, 37.0%) compared with HIV-negative participants (6/99, 6.1%, Chi^2 = 18.098, df = 1, p < 0.001). Most sulfamethoxazole-trimethoprim resistance isolates were ST8 (12/16, 75%), others being ST80, ST25 and ST152. Of the sixteen sulfamethoxazole/trimethoprim resistant isolates only one was *pvl*-positive and none carried the *tsst-1* gene.

2.6. Prevalence of MDR S. aureus

A total of 34/126 (27.0% (95%CI 20.0–35.3%) isolates were multidrug resistant from the VITEK 2 results. The proportion of MDR isolates was higher in isolates from HIV-positive (9/27, 33.3%) than in isolates from HIV-negative participants (25/99, 25.3%), although this was not statistically significant (Chi^2 = 0.683, df = 1, p = 0.409). The most common resistance combination was trimethoprim, penicillin, and tetracycline, observed in 82.4% (28/34) of MDR isolates and accounting for 22.2% (28/126) of all *S. aureus* isolates (Figure 1). There was no significant difference between isolates demonstrating the resistance pattern of trimethoprim, penicillin and tetracycline from HIV-negative (8/27, 29.6%) versus HIV-positive participants (20/99, 20.2%) (Chi^2 = 1.076, df = 1, p = 0.230). There was no significant difference in the proportion of carriage of MDR isolates between groups with recent and no recent antibiotic use (8/25, 32.0% versus 26/101, 25.7%) (Chi^2 = 0.401, df = 1, p = 0.527).

MDR isolates were predominantly ST8 (26.5%, 9/34) and ST80 (7/34, 20.6%). MDR isolates were less frequently *pvl* positive (9/34, 26.5%) than non-MDR isolates (45/92, 48.9%) (Chi^2 = 5.046, df = 1, p = 0.025). Of the MDR isolates, 8.8% (3/34) were positive for *tsst-1* compared to 13.0% (12/92) of the non-MDR isolates (Chi^2 = 0.415, df = 1, p = 0.519).

Highly resistant MDR *S. aureus* that were resistant to at least five antibiotic classes were isolated from one HIV-positive and three HIV-negative participants.

2.7. Prevalence of Genotypic Antibiotic Resistance in MSSA and MRSA Strains

The most common resistance genes detected were beta-lactamase resistance gene *blaZ* (123/126, 96.9%); trimethoprim resistance gene *dfrG* (78/126, 61.9%), and tetracycline resistance gene *tetK* (32/126, 25.4%). Other resistance genes detected included *dfrA* (4/126, 3.2%), *tetM* (1/126, 0.8%), erythromycin resistance gene *ermC* (4/126, 3.2%), and gentamicin resistance gene *aacA-aphD* (2/126, 1.6%). HIV-positive individuals were significantly more frequently colonized by *S. aureus* harboring *dfrA* and *dfrG* genes (22/27, 81.5%) compared to HIV-negative persons (60/99, 60.6%; $Chi^2 = 4.045$, df = 1, $p = 0.044$). There was no significant difference prevalence of *tetK* and *tetM* genes between HIV-positive participants (9/27, 33.3%) compared to HIV-negative persons (24/99, 24.2%; ($Chi^2 = 0.902$, df = 1, $p = 0.342$).

There was almost 100% agreement between phenotypic and genotypic resistance patterns for benzylpenicillin (121/123, 98.4%), trimethoprim (81/82, 98.8%), tetracycline (31/33 93.9%), erythromycin (4/4, 100%), and gentamicin (2/2, 100%). However, there was discrepancy between the MRSA isolates identified by the presence of *mecA* gene ($n = 3$) and those demonstrating oxacillin resistance ($n = 1/3$, 33.3%) and cefoxitin resistance ($n = 2/3$, 66.6%).

3. Discussion

This study described the nasal carriage of *S. aureus* in abattoir workers in western Kenya. The overall nasal carriage of *S. aureus* in this population was 16.0% where 15.6% were MSSA and 0.4% were MRSA. Humans are asymptomatically colonized with nasal *S. aureus* in the range of between 20–30% [40] with MRSA colonization varying between studies and dictated by the methodology used [41]. The carriage of *S. aureus* in this population was lower than expected but consistent with another study conducted in abattoir workers in Nigeria where the prevalence of *S. aureus* carriage was 13.5% [42].

The study population was made up of two groups: HIV-positive abattoir workers and HIV-negative abattoir workers which had an impact on the phenotypes and genotypes of *S. aureus* isolates in this population. The prevalence of HIV infection in this population (12%) was higher than the national average (5%). The reasons for the increased HIV positivity in this population may be related to the sociodemographic group but this was not explored further in this study. The prevalence of *S. aureus* nasal carriage of HIV-positive abattoir workers was significantly higher, 27.0%, when compared to HIV-negative abattoir workers, 14.5%. HIV infection is considered a risk factor for *S. aureus* colonization [22]. This difference in nasal carriage has been reported in previous studies in Africa. In Lagos, Nigeria, HIV-positive study participants were more likely to be colonised with *S. aureus* (33%) compared to HIV-negative participants (21%) [43]. These findings in the sub-Saharan region, suggest that HIV individuals are predisposed to *S. aureus* nasal colonization. Nasal colonization can lead to opportunistic infection in immunocompromised people, and the infection can be life-threatening if not treated promptly [2,44]. This highlights the need to monitor AMR in this population to determine treatment options and improve antimicrobial stewardship.

There was a high proportion of toxigenic strains of *S. aureus* carrying the *pvl* gene (42.9%) and the *tsst-1* gene (11.9%). This is consistent with other studies conducted in sub-Saharan Africa where the carriage of *pvl* genes (33%) is higher than that reported in Europe (5%) [22]. The majority of *pvl* positive strains were ST152-MSSA, which is one of the predominant *pvl*-positive clones in Africa [22,36,45]. The carriage of *pvl*-positive *S. aureus* puts abattoir workers at risk of opportunistic deep skin and soft tissue infections [36,46,47]. The carriage of *S. aureus pvl*-positive strains was not significantly different between HIV-positive abattoir workers (37.0%) and HIV-negative abattoir workers (44.4%) which is consistent with reports from Nigeria, where the proportion of *S. aureus pvl*-positive strains were evenly distributed between isolates from HIV-positive and HIV-negative individuals [43].

There was an inverse relationship between *pvl* carriage and AMR, with 26.5% of MDR isolates being *pvl* positive compared to non-MDR isolates (48.9%) ($p = 0.025$). This differs from other studies in the region where *pvl* carriage has been associated with MDR. An association between *pvl* carriage and sulfamethoxazole/trimethoprim resistance has been observed in Gabon and Nigeria among HIV-positive individuals [43,46].

The prevalence of MRSA carriage (0.4%) identified in this study was low compared to studies conducted with abattoir workers in Europe (5.6%) [48], and the USA 3.6% [16]. However, our results are consistent with other reports of MRSA carriage in Kenya (0.8%) [26] but much lower than studies of MRSA cultured from hospital patients in Kenya (53.4%) [49]. This may suggest that MRSA infection in Kenya is predominantly linked to the hospital environment rather than acquired from the community. The three MRSA isolates belonged to ST88, which is referred to as the "African" community-associated (CA-MRSA) clone [50] but is not the most reported MRSA sequence type in Kenya, which is ST239 [24]. ST88 has been reported in pigs and workers in a Nigerian abattoir and may indicate an animal source [51]. Antimicrobial use in animals is not regulated in Kenya and the most frequently used antibiotics in animals in western Kenya are oxytetracycline and penicillin-streptomycin [52]. Further work to understand MRSA carriage in animals, as well as spread in the human population and environment, is required.

The findings from this study supported prior evidence of *S. aureus* resistance to penicillin, tetracycline, and sulfamethoxazole/trimethoprim in the sub-Saharan region [22]. The proportion of isolates that were phenotypically resistant to penicillin (97.6%), tetracycline (26.2%), and sulfamethoxazole/trimethoprim (12.7%) was consistent with previous studies from Kenya reporting marked resistance to penicillin (76–100%) and moderate resistance to tetracycline (15–20%) and sulfamethoxazole/trimethoprim (30–40%) [25,26]. There was increased frequency of sulfamethoxazole/trimethoprim resistance in HIV-positive abattoir workers (37%) compared to HIV-negative workers (6.1%) ($p < 0.001$), with the majority of resistant strains belonging to ST8-MSSA.

There was high genotype-phenotype concordance between resistance genes detected and antimicrobial susceptibility test (AST) results for most antimicrobials as has been previously reported [25]. However, there were two *mecA* positive MRSA strains that were susceptible to oxacillin and one of these was also susceptible to cefoxitin. This may be due to a misclassification error, although the sensitivity of the VITEK 2 instrument for detecting oxacillin resistance is high (97.5%) [53]. Alternatively, this may indicate oxacillin susceptible *mecA* MRSA (OS-MRSA) strains are circulating in this environment. OS-MRSA strains have previously been identified in other parts of Africa mainly associated with ST88 as described here [54]. Information regarding the presence of the *mecC* gene in these isolates was not available. The presence of OS-MRSA in this setting may complicate treatment options that are based solely on AST results, since OS-MRSA may be misidentified as MSSA, and these isolates can develop β-lactam resistance following antibiotic therapy [55].

Sulfamethoxazole/trimethoprim is an effective antibiotic combination in the treatment and prevention of bacterial infections in people who are HIV positive and has been used to treat *Pneumocystis jiroveci* pneumonia and other bacterial infections in severely immunocompromised HIV-positive individuals. The prophylactic use of sulfamethoxazole/trimethoprim in all HIV-positive individuals regardless of CD4 counts, especially in regions having high prevalence of malaria and/or severe bacterial infections, such as sub-Saharan region [56], may have resulted in the high prevalence of sulfamethoxazole/trimethoprim resistant *S. aureus* in Africa [43,46]. This, coupled with the extensive use of penicillin and tetracycline for use in animal production for both therapeutic and non-therapeutic purposes in Africa [12], has created a favorable environment for the emergence of multidrug resistance *S. aureus* through antibiotic related selective pressure [57,58]. These MDR *S. aureus* reduce the treatment options for effective treatment for HIV-positive individuals with opportunistic infections. With the presence of MDR *S. aureus* that are resistant to additional multiple resistant combinations, including erythromycin, clindamycin, ciprofloxacin and gentamicin, the treatment options will be further diminished and become more expensive. The improved availability of antiretroviral therapy (ART) in sub-Saharan Africa, has led to reduction of severely immune compromised

HIV-positive individuals and fewer cases of serious *Pneumocystis jiroveci* pneumonia and opportunistic infections among HIV-positive individuals [59]. Improved health outcomes for HIV-positive individuals through access to ART may lead to reduced prophylactic use of sulfmethoxazole/trimethoprim in this region. This will aid in the preservation of therapeutic advantages of this affordable drug in treatment and prevention of bacterial infections.

Multi-drug resistant *S. aureus* strains colonizing HIV-positive abattoir workers may be a risk for SSTI since 25% of workers reported being injured at work [60]. MDR *S. aureus* could also be transmitted to the community directly or through the meat supply chain to consumers [4]. In addition, if the respective abattoir workers are hospitalized, the strains can be spread to hospital staff and compromised inpatients, threatening effective treatment of resultant infections [61]. Thus, MDR *S. aureus*-colonized abattoir workers pose a public health problem in hospitals, community, and food industry in Busia County, which can extend to other parts of Kenya and neighboring countries of Kenya since Busia is a border town.

There is a need for increased monitoring of antibiotic usage and surveillance measures for AMR bacteria in both animals and humans in this region already burdened by HIV/AIDS infection and where there is rapidly increasing demand for meat products caused by population growth and urbanization [12]. Additionally, there is a need for strategies to promote the prudent use of antimicrobials and antimicrobial stewardship as described by the global strategy [62]. It is particularly important to strategize on the appropriate use of sulfamethoxazole/trimethoprim, tetracyclines and penicillin in human and animal healthcare and food production in sub-Saharan region, since there were high proportions of resistant isolates to these antimicrobials. It has been demonstrated that a reduction of antibiotic consumption leads to decreased prevalence of antimicrobial resistance [63]. This can be done through national action plans for the prevention and containment of AMR with contributions from human and animal health agencies [39].

There was a delay between the collection of samples and the publication of these findings which may limit the usefulness of these results. However, given the lack of available data regarding the circulating MSSA and MRSA strains and antimicrobial resistance profiles of *S. aureus* in this population the data is a valuable contribution to knowledge regarding AMR in the region and may prove a useful baseline for comparison to future studies. Data regarding the circulating MSSA and MRSA strains in livestock was not available at the time of this publication. This information would have been useful to understand the potential for transmission of isolates between livestock and workers and is a data gap that should be targeted in future research.

4. Materials and Methods

4.1. Study Site

The study area was a 45 km radius from Busia town including most of Busia County, and parts of Bungoma, Siaya and Kakamega Counties spanning the 3200 km^2 of the Lake Victoria ecosystem. The predominant industry in the study area is subsistence agriculture [64]. A census of all abattoirs (n = 156) was conducted in the study area in 2012. Fourteen abattoirs declined to participate. Participants were recruited from 142 abattoirs, 84 ruminants and 58 porcine [60].

4.2. Study Population

A total of 738 abattoir workers were recruited into the study between February and November 2012 from a total of 1005 workers (73.3%) in the selected slaughterhouses. In abattoirs with 12 workers or less all consenting workers were recruited and in abattoirs with more than 12 workers a random selection of twelve workers were recruited [60].

4.3. Data and Sample Collection

All participants were informed of the project objectives and protocol by a clinical officer who collected signed informed consent. Data was collected using a structured questionnaire regarding demographic details, health events and recent antimicrobial use. Nasal samples were collected by rotating a sterile swab five times in both anterior nares, from consenting abattoir workers. The swabs were inoculated in tryptone soya broth with 6% salt and transported in cool boxes to the laboratory for culturing.

Blood was collected by a clinical officer into 4 mL EDTA vacutainers using a butterfly catheter (BD Vacutainer® Safety-Lok™ blood collection set). Samples were transported in cool boxes to the laboratory in Busia. Whole blood samples were stored frozen at −40 °C until transportation to the International Livestock Research Institute (ILRI) laboratory in Nairobi for long term storage at −80 °C. HIV testing was performed on whole blood using the SD Bioline HIV 1/2 Fast 3.0 test strips (Standard Diagnostics Inc., Suwon-si, South Korea).

Swabs were streaked onto Mannitol Salt agar and incubated at 37 °C in air overnight. Suspect *S. aureus* isolates, those fermenting mannitol and producing yellow colonies, were stocked in tryptone soya broth with 10% glycerol and stored at −40 °C and transported on dry ice to Nairobi. Presumptive *S. aureus* isolates were further cultured onto mannitol salt agar (MSA) and sub-cultured to obtain pure culture. The *S. aureus* isolates were identified using Gram reaction (Gram-positive cocci in clumps), catalase, coagulase (tube method using rabbit plasma) and DNase tests. Initially, a long sweep of the colonies was done to allow preservation of genetic diversity of nasal carriage of the participant. During whole genome sequencing, some samples were shown to consist of mixed isolates and these samples were recultured to select single colonies for sequencing and antimicrobial susceptibility testing.

4.4. Phenotypic Antimicrobial Susceptibility Testing

Antimicrobial susceptibility testing (AST) was performed using the VITEK 2 instrument (bioMerieux, Marcy-l'Étoile, France), for 20 antimicrobials including: benzylpenicillin, cefoxitin, oxacillin, ciprofloxacin, erythromycin, chloramphenicol, daptomycin, fusidic acid, gentamicin, linezolid, mupirocin, nitrofurantoin, rifampicin, teicoplanin, tetracycline, tigecycline, trimethoprim, vancomycin, clindamycin, and inducible resistance to clindamycin. The Vitek 2 system uses fluorescence, turbidity and colormetric methods to monitor bacterial growth and uses this to calculate minimum inhibitory concentrations (MICs) [65].

Additionally, due to the clinical importance, antimicrobial resistance to sulfamethoxazole/trimethoprim was tested using the Kirby-Bauer disc diffusion using Clinical and Laboratory Standards Institute (CLSI) guidelines (1.25 + 23.75 µg; TMP/SXT). Zone diameter interpretive standards were: sensitive ≥16 mm, intermediate 11–15 mm and resistant 10 ≤ [66].

Multi-drug resistant *S. aureus* were defined as isolates that were resistant to three or more different antimicrobials using the VITEK results [67–69]. Isolates resistant to 5 or more antimicrobials were described as highly multi-drug resistant.

4.5. Molecular Genotyping

DNA extraction from *S. aureus* isolates was performed using QIAGEN DNeasy Blood & Tissue kit (QIAGEN, Valencia, CA, USA). Staphylococcal cassette chromosome (SCC) *mec* typing were performed using previously described methods [70]. Isolates with the *mecA* gene were classified as MRSA. Panton-Valentine Leukocidin (*pvl*) and toxic shock syndrome toxin-1 (*tsst-1*) gene detection was done by PCR using previously described oligonucleotide primers [71,72] at the Kenya Medical Research Institute Laboratories (KEMRI), Nairobi, Kenya.

DNA extraction from *S. aureus* isolates was performed on a QIAcube, using the QIAamp 96 HT kit (QIAGEN). Genomic libraries were generated and sequenced on an Illumina HiSeq 2000 (Illumina Inc., San Diego, CA, USA) at the Wellcome Sanger Institute, Hinxton, UK. Illumina reads were analysed based on the *S. aureus* MLST database (https://pubmlst.org/organisms/staphylococcus-aureus, accessed on 31 March 2021) [73], and analysis of virulence and antimicrobial resistance genes were conducted using virulence finder database (https://cge.cbs.dtu.dk/services/, accessed on 31 March 2021).

4.6. Genomic Analyses

Paired-end Illumina reads were mapped to the *S. aureus* reference genome ST22 strain HO 5096 0412 (accession number HE681097) using Snippy v4.6.0 (https://github.com/tseemann/snippy, accessed on 31 October 2022). Whole-genome alignments were created by keeping a version of the reference genome with only substitution variants replaced (i.e., SNPs but not indels) using Snippy's *.consensus.subs.fa* output files. The *S. aureus* species core-genome had been previously derived [74] from a collection of 800 *S. aureus* from multiple host species [75]. The portion of the reference genome (2.83 Mb) corresponding to the core genome (1.76 Mb) was kept from whole-genome alignments and used to generate maximum likelihood trees using IQ-TREE v1.6.10 with default settings. The resulting core-genome phylogeny was plotted with isolate metadata using ggtree v.3.0.4 [76] and ggtreeExtra v.1.2.3 on R v4.1.0 [77].

4.7. Statistical Analyses

Statistical analysis was performed using the chi-squared test. A p-value <0.05 was considered an indication of significant difference.

4.8. Ethical Approval

The study was approved by the Centre for Microbiology Research Centre Scientific Committee, Kenya Medical Research Institute scientific steering Committee and Ethical Review Committee (SSC No 2086 granted 31 October 2011 and 2944 granted 13 May 2015).

5. Conclusions

This study identifies the circulating MSSA and MRSA strains in a population occupationally exposed to livestock in rural western Kenya. This gives an improved understanding of the epidemiology of *S. aureus* particularly the strains, sources, and risk groups in a setting that has not been previously studied. More importantly, the study indicates the levels of AMR and prevalence of toxigenic genes in *S. aureus* isolates, which is particularly important in this community with high prevalence of immunocompromised individuals. This information can contribute to developing measures for the prevention and containment of AMR.

Supplementary Materials: The following supporting information can be downloaded at: https://www.mdpi.com/article/10.3390/antibiotics11121726/s1, Table S1: Sequence types of MSSA and MRSA strains isolated from nasal of HIV positive and negative abattoir workers Busia County.

Author Contributions: Conceptualization, B.A.O. and E.A.J.C.; Data curation, B.A.O., F.C., E.M.H. and E.A.J.C.; Formal analysis, B.A.O., R.N., B.B., F.C., E.M.H. and E.A.J.C.; Funding acquisition, E.M.F., S.-H.W., W.G., S.J.P. and E.A.J.C.; Investigation, B.A.O., E.M.H. and E.A.J.C.; Methodology, B.A.O., C.L.G., E.M.F., E.M.H., S.K. and E.A.J.C.; Resources, E.M.F. and S.J.P.; Supervision, L.B., G.G., W.O., S.-H.W., W.G. and S.K.; Writing—original draft, B.A.O.; Writing—review and editing, C.L.G., S.-H.W., E.M.H., S.J.P. and E.A.J.C. All authors have read and agreed to the published version of the manuscript.

Funding: Benear Obanda's research was supported in part by One Health Eastern Africa Research Training (OHEART) program, at the Ohio State University, Global One Health initiative (GOHi) through the financial support from National Institutes of Health (NIH) Fogarty International Center (grant number D43TW008650) awarded to GW and SHW. EAJC was supported with an Innovation Initiative Grant (GR000154) from the University of Edinburgh, and Medical Research Council grants (1525363 and 971282). A Wellcome Trust grant (085308) was awarded to EMF and supported the People and their Zoonoses project (PAZ). Support was received from the CGIAR Research Program on Agriculture for Nutrition and Health (A4NH), led by the International Food Policy Research Institute (IFPRI). We acknowledge the CGIAR Fund Donors (https://www.cgiar.org/funders/, accessed on 31 October 2022). This work was also supported by the Health Innovation Challenge Fund (WT098600,

HICF-T5-342), a parallel funding partnership between the Department of Health and Wellcome Trust. The views expressed in this publication are those of the author(s) and not necessarily those of the Department of Health or Wellcome Trust." and "The APC was funded by the University of Liverpool".

Institutional Review Board Statement: The study was conducted in accordance with the Declaration of Helsinki, and approved by the Institutional Review Board (or Ethics Committee) of the Centre for Microbiology Research Centre Scientific Committee, Kenya Medical Research Institute scientific steering Committee and Ethical Review Committee (SSC No 2086 granted on 31 October 2011 and 2944 granted on 13 May 2015).

Informed Consent Statement: Informed consent was obtained from all subjects involved in the study.

Data Availability Statement: Data is contained within the article and Supplementary Material.

Acknowledgments: Thank you to the PAZ team—Hannah Kariuki, John Mwaniki, James Akoko, Omoto Lazarus, Fred Amanya, Lorren Alumasa, Daniel Cheruyoit, Isaac Obara, Dominic Njuguna, Abraham Simiyu, Gideon Maloba, George Omondi, Lillian Abonyo, and Bartholomew Wabwire for their hard work and diligence. We are grateful to all the participating slaughterhouse workers for their willingness to be involved in the research, and the national and local veterinary authorities for their collaboration.

Conflicts of Interest: The authors declare no conflict of interest. The funders had no role in the design of the study; in the collection, analyses, or interpretation of data; in the writing of the manuscript; or in the decision to publish the results.

References

1. Williams, R.E. Healthy carriage of *Staphylococcus aureus*: Its prevalence and importance. *Bacteriol. Rev.* **1963**, *27*, 56–71. [CrossRef] [PubMed]
2. Sakr, A.; Brégeon, F.; Mège, J.L.; Rolain, J.M.; Blin, O. *Staphylococcus aureus* nasal colonization: An update on mechanisms, epidemiology, risk factors, and subsequent infections. *Front. Microbiol.* **2018**, *9*, 2419. [CrossRef] [PubMed]
3. Wertheim, H.F.L.; Melles, D.C.; Vos, M.C.; van Leeuwen, W.; van Belkum, A.; Verbrugh, H.A.; Nouwen, J.L. The role of nasal carriage in *Staphylococcus aureus* infections. *Lancet Infect. Dis.* **2005**, *5*, 751–762. [CrossRef]
4. Velasco, V.; Quezada-Aguiluz, M.; Bello-Toledo, H. *Staphylococcus aureus* in the Meat Supply Chain: Detection Methods, Antimicrobial Resistance, and Virulence Factors. In *Staphylococcus and Streptococcus*; Kırmusaoğlu, S., Ed.; IntechOpen: Rijeka, Croatia, 2019.
5. Hidron, A.; Moanna, M.D.A.; Russell Kempker, M.D.; David Rimland, M.D. Methicillin-resistant *Staphylococcus aureus* in HIV-infected patients. *Infect. Drug Resist.* **2010**, *73*, 73–86. [CrossRef] [PubMed]
6. NACC. *Kenya HIV Estimates Report 2018*; National AIDS Control Council: Nairobi, Kenya, 2018.
7. Ministry of Health. *National Manual for the Management of HIV-Related Opportunistic Infections and Conditions*; Ojoo, S., Ed.; Ministry of Health: Nairobi, Kenya, 2008. Available online: http://guidelines.health.go.ke:8000/media/National_Manual_for_the_management_of_HIV_related_OIs.pdf (accessed on 23 October 2022).
8. Dworkin, M.S.; Williamson, J.; Jones, J.L.; Kaplan, J.E. Prophylaxis with Trimethoprim-Sulfamethoxazole for Human Immunodeficiency Virus—Infected Patients: Impact on Risk for Infectious Diseases. *Clin. Infect. Dis.* **2001**, *60601*, 393–398. [CrossRef] [PubMed]
9. Fair, R.J.; Tor, Y. Antibiotics and bacterial resistance in the 21st century. *Perspect. Medicin. Chem.* **2014**, *6*, 25–64. [CrossRef] [PubMed]
10. Martin, J.N.; Rose, D.A.; Hadley, W.K.; Perdreau-Remington, F.; Lam, P.K.; Gerberding, J.L. Emergence of Trimethoprim-Sulfamethoxazole Resistance in the AIDS Era. *J. Infect. Dis.* **1999**, *180*, 1809–1818. [CrossRef]
11. Murray, C.J.; Ikuta, K.S.; Sharara, F.; Swetschinski, L.; Robles Aguilar, G.; Gray, A.; Han, C.; Bisignano, C.; Rao, P.; Wool, E.; et al. Global burden of bacterial antimicrobial resistance in 2019: A systematic analysis. *Lancet* **2022**, *399*, 629–655. [CrossRef]
12. Kimera, Z.I.; Mshana, S.E.; Rweyemamu, M.M.; Mboera, L.E.G.; Matee, M.I.N. Antimicrobial use and resistance in food-producing animals and the environment: An African perspective. *Antimicrob. Resist. Infect. Control* **2020**, *9*, 37. [CrossRef]
13. Dweba, C.C.; Zishiri, O.T.; El Zowalaty, M.E. Methicillin-resistant staphylococcus aureus: Livestock-associated, antimicrobial, and heavy metal resistance. *Infect. Drug Resist.* **2018**, *11*, 2497–2509. [CrossRef]
14. Waters, A.E.; Contente-Cuomo, T.; Buchhagen, J.; Liu, C.M.; Watson, L.; Pearce, K.; Foster, J.T.; Bowers, J.; Driebe, E.M.; Engelthaler, D.M.; et al. Multidrug-resistant staphylococcus aureus in US meat and poultry. *Clin. Infect. Dis.* **2011**, *52*, 1227–1230. [CrossRef] [PubMed]
15. Van Loo, I.; Huijsdens, X.; Tiemersma, E.; De Neeling, A.; Van De Sande-Bruinsma, N.; Beaujean, D.; Voss, A.; Kluytmans, J. Emergence of methicillin-resistant *Staphylococcus aureus* of animal origin in humans. *Emerg. Infect. Dis.* **2007**, *13*, 1834–1839. [CrossRef] [PubMed]

16. Leibler, J.H.; Jordan, J.A.; Brownstein, K.; Lander, L.; Price, L.B.; Perry, M.J. *Staphylococcus aureus* nasal carriage among beefpacking workers in a Midwestern United States slaughterhouse. *PLoS ONE* **2016**, *11*, e0148789. [CrossRef] [PubMed]
17. Ivbule, M.; Miklaševičs, E.; Čupane, L.; Berziņa, L.; Baliņš, A.; Valdovska, A. Presence of methicillin-resistant *Staphylococcus aureus* in slaughterhouse environment, pigs, carcasses, and workers. *J. Vet. Res.* **2017**, *61*, 267–277. [CrossRef]
18. Van Rijen, M.M.L.; Bosch, T.; Verkade, E.J.M.; Schouls, L.; Kluytmans, J.A.J.W. Livestock-associated MRSA carriage in patients without direct contact with livestock. *PLoS ONE* **2014**, *9*, e100294. [CrossRef]
19. Larsen, J.; Petersen, A.; Sørum, M.; Stegger, M.; van Alphen, L.; Valentiner-Branth, P.; Knudsen, L.K.; Larsen, L.S.; Feingold, B.; Price, L.B.; et al. Meticillin-resistant *Staphylococcus aureus* CC398 is an increasing cause of disease in people with no livestock contact in Denmark, 1999 to 2011. *Eurosurveillance* **2015**, *20*, 30021. [CrossRef]
20. Enright, M.C.; Day, N.P.J.; Davies, C.E.; Peacock, S.J.; Spratt, B.G. Multilocus sequence typing for characterization of methicillin-resistant and methicillin-susceptible clones of *Staphylococcus aureus*. *J. Clin. Microbiol.* **2000**, *38*, 1008–1015. [CrossRef]
21. Enright, M.C.; Robinson, D.A.; Randle, G.; Feil, E.J.; Grundmann, H.; Spratt, B.G. The evolutionary history of methicillin-resistant *Staphylococcus aureus* (MRSA). *Proc. Natl. Acad. Sci. USA* **2002**, *99*, 7687–7692. [CrossRef]
22. Schaumburg, F.; Alabi, A.S.; Peters, G.; Becker, K. New epidemiology of *Staphylococcus aureus* infection in Africa. *Clin. Microbiol. Infect. Off. Publ. Eur. Soc. Clin. Microbiol. Infect. Dis.* **2014**, *20*, 589–596. [CrossRef]
23. Lawal, O.U.; Ayobami, O.; Abouelfetouh, A.; Mourabit, N.; Kaba, M.; Egyir, B.; Abdulgader, S.M.; Shittu, A.O. A 6-Year Update on the Diversity of Methicillin-Resistant *Staphylococcus aureus* Clones in Africa: A Systematic Review. *Front. Microbiol.* **2022**, *13*, 860436. [CrossRef]
24. Nyasinga, J.; Omuse, G.; John, N.; Nyerere, A.; Abdulgader, S.; Newton, M.; Whitelaw, A.; Revathi, G. Epidemiology of *Staphylococcus aureus* Infections in Kenya: Current State, Gaps and Opportunities. *Open J. Med. Microbiol.* **2020**, *10*, 204–221. [CrossRef]
25. Kyany'a, C.; Nyasinga, J.; Matano, D.; Oundo, V.; Wacira, S.; Sang, W.; Musila, L. Phenotypic and genotypic characterization of clinical Staphylococcus aureus isolates from Kenya. *BMC Microbiol.* **2019**, *19*, 245. [CrossRef] [PubMed]
26. Aiken, A.M.; Mutuku, I.M.; Sabat, A.J.; Akkerboom, V.; Mwangi, J.; Scott, J.A.G.; Morpeth, S.C.; Friedrich, A.W.; Grundmann, H. Carriage of *Staphylococcus aureus* in Thika Level 5 Hospital, Kenya: A cross-sectional study. *Antimicrob. Resist. Infect. Control* **2014**, *3*, 22. [CrossRef] [PubMed]
27. Omuse, G.; Zyl, K.N.; Hoek, K.; Abdulgader, S.; Kariuki, S.; Whitelaw, A.; Revathi, G. Molecular characterization of *Staphylococcus aureus* isolates from various healthcare institutions in Nairobi, Kenya: A cross sectional study. *Ann. Clin. Microbiol. Antimicrob.* **2016**, *15*, 51. [CrossRef]
28. Nyasinga, J.; Kyany'a, C.; Okoth, R.; Oundo, V.; Matano, D.; Wacira, S.; Sang, W.; Musembi, S.; Musila, L. A six-member SNP assay on the iPlex MassARRAY platform provides a rapid and affordable alternative for typing major African *Staphylococcus aureus* types. *Access Microbiol.* **2019**, *1*, e000018. [CrossRef]
29. McCormick, J.K.; Yarwood, J.M.; Schlievert, P.M. Toxic shock syndrome and bacterial superantigens: An update. *Annu. Rev. Microbiol.* **2001**, *55*, 77–104. [CrossRef] [PubMed]
30. Dinges, M.M.; Orwin, P.M.; Schlievert, P.M. Exotoxins of *Staphylococcus aureus*. *Clin. Microbiol. Rev.* **2000**, *13*, 16–34. [CrossRef]
31. McGrath, B.; Rutledge, F.; Broadfield, E. Necrotising Pneumonia, *Staphylococcus Aureus* and Panton-Valentine Leukocidin. *J. Intensive Care Soc.* **2008**, *9*, 170–172. [CrossRef]
32. Shallcross, L.J.; Fragaszy, E.; Johnson, A.M.; Hayward, A.C. The role of the Panton-Valentine leucocidin toxin in staphylococcal disease: A systematic review and meta-analysis. *Lancet Infect. Dis.* **2013**, *13*, 43–54. [CrossRef]
33. Voyich, J.M.; Otto, M.; Mathema, B.; Braughton, K.R.; Whitney, A.R.; Welty, D.; Long, R.D.; Dorward, D.W.; Gardner, D.J.; Lina, G.; et al. Is Panton-Valentine leukocidin the major virulence determinant in community-associated methicillin-resistant *Staphylococcus aureus* disease? *J. Infect. Dis.* **2006**, *194*, 1761–1770. [CrossRef]
34. Labandeira-Rey, M.; Couzon, F.; Boisset, S.; Brown, E.L.; Bes, M.; Benito, Y.; Barbu, E.M.; Vazquez, V.; Höök, M.; Etienne, J.; et al. *Staphylococcus aureus* Panton-Valentine leukocidin causes necrotizing pneumonia. *Science* **2007**, *315*, 1130–1133. [CrossRef] [PubMed]
35. Gillet, Y.; Issartel, B.; Vanhems, P.; Fournet, J.-C.; Lina, G.; Bes, M.; Vandenesch, F.; Piémont, Y.; Brousse, N.; Floret, D.; et al. Association between *Staphylococcus aureus* strains carrying gene for Panton-Valentine leukocidin and highly lethal necrotising pneumonia in young immunocompetent patients. *Lancet* **2002**, *359*, 753–759. [CrossRef] [PubMed]
36. Breurec, S.; Zriouil, S.B.; Fall, C.; Boisier, P.; Brisse, S.; Djibo, S.; Etienne, J.; Fonkoua, M.C.; Perrier-Gros-Claude, J.D.; Pouillot, R.; et al. Epidemiology of methicillin-resistant *Staphylococcus aureus* lineages in five major African towns: Emergence and spread of atypical clones. *Clin. Microbiol. Infect.* **2011**, *17*, 160–165. [CrossRef] [PubMed]
37. Holmes, A.; Ganner, M.; McGuane, S.; Pitt, T.L.; Cookson, B.D.; Kearns, A.M. *Staphylococcus aureus* isolates carrying panton-valentine leucocidin genes in England and Wales: Frequency, characterization, and association with clinical disease. *J. Clin. Microbiol.* **2005**, *43*, 2384–2390. [CrossRef]
38. Adesiyun, A.A.; Lenz, W.; Schaal, K.P. Production of toxic shock syndrome toxin-1 (TSST-1) by *Staphylococcus aureus* strains isolated from humans, animals and foods in Nigeria. *Microbiologica* **1992**, *15*, 125–133. [PubMed]
39. GoK. National Policy for the Prevention and Containment of Antimicrobial Resistance, Nairobi, Kenya: Government of Kenya, April 2017. 2017. Available online: https://www.health.go.ke/wp-content/uploads/2017/04/Kenya-AMR-Containment-Policy-_Final_April.pdf (accessed on 23 October 2022).

40. Lucia Preoţescu, L.; Streinu-Cercel, O. Prevalence of nasal carriage of S aureus in children. *Germs* **2013**, *3*, 49–51. [CrossRef]
41. Hassoun, A.; Linden, P.K.; Friedman, B. Incidence, prevalence, and management of MRSA bacteremia across patient populations-a review of recent developments in MRSA management and treatment. *Crit. Care* **2017**, *21*, 211. [CrossRef]
42. Odetokun, I.A.; Ballhausen, B.; Adetunji, V.O.; Ghali-Mohammed, I.; Adelowo, M.T.; Adetunji, S.A.; Fetsch, A. *Staphylococcus aureus* in two municipal abattoirs in Nigeria: Risk perception, spread and public health implications. *Vet. Microbiol.* **2018**, *216*, 52–59. [CrossRef]
43. Olalekan, A.O.; Schaumburg, F.; Nurjadi, D.; Dike, A.E.; Ojurongbe, O.; Kolawole, D.O.; Kun, J.F.; Zanger, P. Clonal expansion accounts for an excess of antimicrobial resistance in *Staphylococcus aureus* colonising HIV-positive individuals in Lagos, Nigeria. *Int. J. Antimicrob. Agents* **2012**, *40*, 268–272. [CrossRef]
44. Nguyen, M.H.; Kauffman, C.A.; Goodman, R.P.; Squier, C.; Arbeit, R.D.; Singh, N.; Wagener, M.M.; Yu, V.L. Nasal carriage of and infection with *Staphylococcus aureus* in HIV-infected patients. *Ann. Intern. Med.* **1999**, *130*, 221–225. [CrossRef]
45. Ouedraogo, A.S.; Dunyach-Remy, C.; Kissou, A.; Sanou, S.; Poda, A.; Kyelem, C.G.; Solassol, J.; Bañuls, A.L.; Van De Perre, P.; Ouédraogo, R.; et al. High nasal carriage rate of *Staphylococcus aureus* containing panton-valentine leukocidin- and EDIN-encoding genes in community and hospital settings in Burkina Faso. *Front. Microbiol.* **2016**, *7*, 1406. [CrossRef] [PubMed]
46. Kraef, C.; Alabi, A.S.; Peters, G.; Becker, K.; Kremsner, P.G.; Rossatanga, E.G.; Mellmann, A.; Grobusch, M.P.; Zanger, P.; Schaumburg, F. Co-detection of Panton-Valentine leukocidin encoding genes and cotrimoxazole resistance in *Staphylococcus aureus* in Gabon: Implications for HIV-patients' care. *Front. Microbiol.* **2015**, *6*, 60. [CrossRef]
47. Vandenesch, F.; Naimi, T.; Enright, M.C.; Lina, G.; Nimmo, G.R.; Heffernan, H.; Liassine, N.; Bes, M.; Greenland, T.; Reverdy, M.E.; et al. Community-acquired methicillin-resistant *staphylococcus aureus* carrying panton-valentine leukocidin genes: Worldwide emergence. *Emerg. Infect. Dis.* **2003**, *9*, 978–984. [CrossRef] [PubMed]
48. Van Cleef, B.A.G.L.; Broens, E.M.; Voss, A.; Huijsdens, X.W.; Züchner, L.; Van Benthem, B.H.B.; Kluytmans, J.A.J.W.; Mulders, M.N.; Van De Giessen, A.W. High prevalence of nasal MRSA carriage in slaughterhouse workers in contact with live pigs in the Netherlands. *Epidemiol. Infect.* **2010**, *138*, 756–763. [CrossRef] [PubMed]
49. Wangai, F.K.; Masika, M.M.; Maritim, M.C.; Seaton, R.A. Methicillin-resistant Staphylococcus aureus (MRSA) in East Africa: Red alert or red herring? *BMC Infect. Dis.* **2019**, *19*, 596. [CrossRef]
50. Kpeli, G.; Buultjens, A.H.; Giulieri, S.; Owusu-Mireku, E.; Aboagye, S.Y.; Baines, S.L.; Seemann, T.; Bulach, D.; da Silva, A.G.; Monk, I.R.; et al. Genomic analysis of ST88 communityacquired methicillin resistant *Staphylococcus aureus* in Ghana. *PeerJ* **2017**, *2017*, 3047. [CrossRef]
51. Odetokun, I.A.; Afolaranmi, Z.M.; Nuhu, A.A.; Borokinni, B.O.; Ghali-Mohammed, I.; Cisse, H.; Alhaji, N.B. Knowledge and self-reported food safety practices among meat consumers in Ilorin, Nigeria. *Dialogues Health* **2022**, *1*, 100039. [CrossRef]
52. Kemp, S.A.; Pinchbeck, G.L.; Fèvre, E.M.; Williams, N.J. A Cross-Sectional Survey of the Knowledge, Attitudes, and Practices of Antimicrobial Users and Providers in an Area of High-Density Livestock-Human Population in Western Kenya. *Front. Vet. Sci.* **2021**, *8*, 1070. [CrossRef]
53. Roisin, S.; Nonhoff, C.; Denis, O.; Struelens, M.J. Evaluation of new Vitek 2 card and disk diffusion method for determining susceptibility of *Staphylococcus aureus* to oxacillin. *J. Clin. Microbiol.* **2008**, *46*, 2525–2528. [CrossRef]
54. Conceição, T.; Coelho, C.; de Lencastre, H.; Aires-de-Sousa, M. Frequent occurrence of oxacillin-susceptible mecA-positive *Staphylococcus aureus* (OS-MRSA) strains in two African countries. *J. Antimicrob. Chemother.* **2015**, *70*, 3200–3204. [CrossRef]
55. Boonsiri, T.; Watanabe, S.; Tan, X.E.; Thitiananpakorn, K.; Narimatsu, R.; Sasaki, K.; Takenouchi, R.; Sato'o, Y.; Aiba, Y.; Kiga, K.; et al. Identification and characterization of mutations responsible for the β-lactam resistance in oxacillin-susceptible mecA-positive *Staphylococcus aureus*. *Sci. Rep.* **2020**, *10*, 16907. [CrossRef] [PubMed]
56. WHO. Guidelines on Post-Exposure Prophylaxis for HIV and the Use of Co-Trimoxazole Prophylaxis for HIV-Related Infections among Adults, Adolescents and Children: Recommendations for a Public Health Approach: Supplement to the 2013 Consolidated Guidelines on th [Internet]. 2014. Available online: https://apps.who.int/iris/handle/10665/145719 (accessed on 23 October 2022).
57. Aslam, B.; Khurshid, M.; Arshad, M.I.; Muzammil, S.; Rasool, M.; Yasmeen, N.; Shah, T.; Chaudhry, T.H.; Rasool, M.H.; Shahid, A.; et al. Antibiotic Resistance: One Health One World Outlook. *Front. Cell. Infect. Microbiol.* **2021**, *11*, 1153. [CrossRef] [PubMed]
58. Marbou, W.J.T.; Kuete, V. Bacterial resistance and immunological profiles in HIV-infected and non-infected patients at Mbouda AD LUCEM Hospital in Cameroon. *J. Infect. Public Health* **2017**, *10*, 269–276. [CrossRef] [PubMed]
59. Günthard, H.F.; Saag, M.S.; Benson, C.A.; Del Rio, C.; Eron, J.J.; Gallant, J.E.; Hoy, J.F.; Mugavero, M.J.; Sax, P.E.; Thompson, M.A.; et al. Antiretroviral drugs for treatment and prevention of HIV infection in Adults: 2016 recommendations of the international antiviral society-USA Panel. *JAMA—J. Am. Med. Assoc.* **2016**, *316*, 191–210. [CrossRef]
60. Cook, E.A.J.; De Glanville, W.A.; Thomas, L.F.; Kariuki, S.; de Clare Bronsvoort, B.M.; Fèvre, E.M. Working conditions and public health risks in slaughterhouses in western Kenya. *BMC Public Health* **2017**, *17*, 14. [CrossRef]
61. Smith, D.L.; Harris, A.D.; Johnson, J.A.; Silbergeld, E.K.; Morris, J.G. Animal antibiotic use has an early but important impact on the emergence of antibiotic resistance in human commensal bacteria. *Proc. Natl. Acad. Sci. USA* **2002**, *99*, 6434–6439. [CrossRef]
62. WHO. *WHO Global Strategy for Containment of Antimicrobial Resistance*; WHO: Geneva, Switzerland, 2001.

63. Seppälä, H.; Klaukka, T.; Vuopio-Varkila, J.; Muotiala, A.; Helenius, H.; Lager, K.; Huovinen, P. The effect of changes in the consumption of macrolide antibiotics on erythromycin resistance in group A streptococci in Finland. Finnish Study Group for Antimicrobial Resistance. *N. Engl. J. Med.* **1997**, *337*, 441–446. [CrossRef]
64. Fèvre, E.M.; de Glanville, W.A.; Thomas, L.F.; Cook, E.A.J.; Kariuki, S.; Wamae, C.N. An integrated study of human and animal infectious disease in the Lake Victoria crescent small-holder crop-livestock production system, Kenya. *BMC Infect. Dis.* **2017**, *17*, 457. [CrossRef]
65. Ligozzi, M.; Bernini, C.; Bonora, M.G.; De Fatima, M.; Zuliani, J.; Fontana, R. Evaluation of the VITEK 2 system for identification and antimicrobial susceptibility testing of medically relevant gram-positive cocci. *J. Clin. Microbiol.* **2002**, *40*, 1681–1686. [CrossRef]
66. CLSI. *Performance Standards for Antimicrobial Sensitivity Testing. CLSI Supplement M100*, 29th ed.; Clinical and Laboratory Standards Institute: Wayne, PA, USA, 2019.
67. Wang, M.; Wei, H.; Zhao, Y.; Shang, L.; Di, L.; Lyu, C.; Liu, J. Analysis of multidrug-resistant bacteria in 3223 patients with hospital-acquired infections (HAI) from a tertiary general hospital in China. *Bosn. J. Basic Med. Sci.* **2019**, *19*, 86–93. [CrossRef]
68. Magiorakos, A.-P.; Srinivasan, A.; Carey, R.B.; Carmeli, Y.; Falagas, M.E.; Giske, C.G.; Harbarth, S.; Hindler, J.F.; Kahlmeter, G.; Olsson-Liljequist, B.; et al. Multidrug-resistant, extensively drug-resistant and pandrug-resistant bacteria: An international expert proposal for interim standard definitions for acquired resistance. *Clin. Microbiol. Infect.* **2012**, *18*, 268–281. [CrossRef] [PubMed]
69. Falagas, M.E.; Koletsi, P.K.; Bliziotis, I.A. The diversity of definitions of multidrug-resistant (MDR) and pandrug-resistant (PDR) *Acinetobacter baumannii* and *Pseudomonas aeruginosa*. *J. Med. Microbiol.* **2006**, *55*, 1619–1629. [CrossRef]
70. Kondo, Y.; Ito, T.; Ma, X.X.; Watanabe, S.; Kreiswirth, B.N.; Etienne, J.; Hiramatsu, K. Combination of multiplex PCRs for staphylococcal cassette chromosome mec type assignment: Rapid identification system for mec, ccr, and major differences in junkyard regions. *Antimicrob. Agents Chemother.* **2007**, *51*, 264–274. [CrossRef]
71. Lina, G.; Piémont, Y.; Godail-Gamot, F.; Bes, M.; Peter, M.O.; Gauduchon, V.; Vandenesch, F.; Etienne, J. Involvement of Panton-Valentine leukocidin-producing *Staphylococcus aureus* in primary skin infections and pneumonia. *Clin. Infect. Dis.* **1999**, *29*, 1128–1132. [CrossRef] [PubMed]
72. Jarraud, S.; Mougel, C.; Thioulouse, J.; Lina, G.; Meugnier, H.; Forey, F.; Nesme, X.; Etienne, J.; Vandenesch, F. Relationships between *Staphylococcus aureus* genetic background, virulence factors, agr groups (alleles), and human disease. *Infect. Immun.* **2002**, *70*, 631–641. [CrossRef] [PubMed]
73. Jolley, K.A.; Bray, J.E.; Maiden, M.C.J. Open-access bacterial population genomics: BIGSdb software, the PubMLST.org website and their applications. *Wellcome Open Res.* **2018**, *3*, 124. [CrossRef]
74. Coll, F.; Raven, K.E.; Knight, G.M.; Blane, B.; Harrison, E.M.; Leek, D.; Enoch, D.A.; Brown, N.M.; Parkhill, J.; Peacock, S.J. Definition of a genetic relatedness cutoff to exclude recent transmission of meticillin-resistant *Staphylococcus aureus*: A genomic epidemiology analysis. *Lancet Microbe* **2020**, *1*, e328–e335. [CrossRef]
75. Richardson, E.J.; Bacigalupe, R.; Harrison, E.M.; Weinert, L.A.; Lycett, S.; Vrieling, M.; Robb, K.; Hoskisson, P.A.; Holden, M.T.G.; Feil, E.J.; et al. Gene exchange drives the ecological success of a multi-host bacterial pathogen. *Nat. Ecol. Evol.* **2018**, *2*, 1468–1478. [CrossRef]
76. Yu, G. Using ggtree to Visualize Data on Tree-Like Structures. *Curr. Protoc. Bioinform.* **2020**, *69*, e96. [CrossRef]
77. Xu, S.; Dai, Z.; Guo, P.; Fu, X.; Liu, S.; Zhou, L.; Tang, W.; Feng, T.; Chen, M.; Zhan, L.; et al. GgtreeExtra: Compact Visualization of Richly Annotated Phylogenetic Data. *Mol. Biol. Evol.* **2021**, *38*, 4039–4042. [CrossRef]

antibiotics

MDPI

Article

Molecular Epidemiology of *Staphylococcus aureus* and MRSA in Bedridden Patients and Residents of Long-Term Care Facilities

Lucas Porangaba Silva [1], Carlos Magno Castelo Branco Fortaleza [2], Nathalia Bibiana Teixeira [1], Luís Thadeo Poianas Silva [1], Carolina Destro de Angelis [1] and Maria de Lourdes Ribeiro de Souza da Cunha [1,*]

1 Department of Chemical and Biological Sciences, Biosciences Institute, UNESP—Universidade Estadual Paulista, Botucatu 18618-691, SP, Brazil
2 Department of Infectology, Dermatology, Diagnostic Imaging and Radiotherapy, Botucatu School of Medicine, UNESP—Universidade Estadual Paulista, Botucatu 18618-970, SP, Brazil
* Correspondence: mlrs.cunha@unesp.br

Abstract: At present, multidrug-resistant microorganisms are already responsible for community-acquired infections. Methicillin-resistant *Staphylococcus aureus* (MRSA) poses a serious public health risk worldwide because of the rapid spread and diversification of pandemic clones that are characterized by increasing virulence and antimicrobial resistance. The aim of this study was to identify the prevalence and factors associated with nasal, oral and rectal carriage of *S. aureus* and MRSA in bedridden patients and residents of long-term care facilities for the elderly (LTCFs) in Botucatu, SP, Brazil. Nasal, oral and rectal swab isolates obtained from 226 LTCF residents or home-bedridden patients between 2017 and 2018 were submitted to susceptibility testing, detection of the *mecA* gene, SCC*mec* characterization, and molecular typing by pulsed-field gel electrophoresis (PFGE) and multilocus sequence typing (MLST). Logistic regression analysis was used to identify risk factors associated with the presence of *S. aureus* and MRSA. The prevalence of *S. aureus* and MRSA was 33.6% (n = 76) and 8% (n = 18), respectively. At the nine LTCFs studied, the prevalence of *S. aureus* ranged from 16.6% to 85.7% and that of MRSA from 13.3% to 25%. Living in an LTCF, male gender, a history of surgeries, and a high Charlson Comorbidity Index score were risk factors associated with *S. aureus* carriage, while MRSA carriage was positively associated with male gender. This study showed a high prevalence of *S. aureus* among elderly residents of small (<15 residents) and medium-sized (15–49 residents) LTCFs and a higher prevalence of MRSA in the oropharynx.

Keywords: elderly population; long-term care facility; bedridden patients; *Staphylococcus aureus*; MRSA; molecular epidemiology

1. Introduction

The epidemiology of *Staphylococcus aureus* has undergone a conceptual revolution over recent decades [1]. This phenomenon was partly due to important changes in the epidemiological behavior of this microorganism [2]. However, old concepts were also reassessed in view of new knowledge arising from clinical and experimental research [3]. Within this context, methicillin-resistant *S. aureus* (MRSA), which have traditionally been addressed as exclusive agents of healthcare-associated [HA] infections, are now being recognized as the causative agent of severe community-acquired disease (community-associated [CA]-MRSA) [4,5].

It is estimated that about 20 to 40% of the world population are asymptomatic nasal *S. aureus* carriers and are, therefore, at increased risk of infection [6]. Colonization is a precursor stage of invasive disease. It is believed that *S. aureus* carriers are more susceptible to acquiring infection and that they are an important source of bacterial dissemination among individuals [7]. Studies have shown that colonized individuals with a high bacterial load have a six-fold higher risk of developing staphylococcal infections than non-carriers or individuals with a low bacterial load [8]. This phenomenon appears to be even more common among carriers of MRSA [9,10].

Furthermore, an important facet of the epidemiology of *S. aureus* is the involvement of "special populations". This term refers to population strata differentiated by ecological pressures and/or specific morbidity conditions, such as elderly people and bedridden individuals. The emergence of MRSA strains poses a special risk to known vulnerable populations. Within this context, two distinct situations are of special interest: institutionalized elderly people living in nursing homes, which represent a link between the community and the hospital, and dependent (bedridden) individuals who are cared for at home and who are intermittently exposed to health services.

Elderly patients have a high morbidity and mortality risk from infectious diseases due to the presence of comorbidities, physical and cognitive disabilities, and declining immunity [11]. The risk is even higher among elderly people who are colonized with *S. aureus*, which can cause severe infection in the presence of associated comorbidities like congestive heart failure, diabetes, lung disease, and kidney failure [12]. These comorbidities are commonly found in bedridden patients cared for at home or residents of long-term care facilities for the elderly (LTCFs). One environment that can promote the acquisition and dissemination of MRSA is precisely the nursing home, where cross-transmission occurs due to permanent living in a confined environment and reduced adherence to hygienic measures as a result of cognitive impairment [13]. This fact puts residents at constant risk of colonization and infection with this microorganism. In addition, the resistance of MRSA to first-line antibiotics such as penicillin poses a risk to immunocompromised patients and makes it more difficult to treat infections [14].

Nursing homes generally admit hospitalized individuals and may therefore become a reservoir of multidrug-resistant microorganisms [15], facilitating the spread from facility to facility and leaving hospitals with low MRSA levels at risk of an outbreak if they do not maintain effective infection control [16]. Although advances in antibiotic therapy have decreased mortality, the prognosis of elderly patients infected with multidrug-resistant bacteria remains the same. Insights into the risk factors associated with the carriage and dissemination of MRSA strains in different groups of elderly people (bedridden and institutionalized) can have significant implications for the treatment and prevention of these infections.

We currently have adequate tools for studying the epidemiology of *S. aureus*, including staphylococcal cassette chromosome (SCC*mec*) typing to identify types that are more prevalent in hospital (SCC*mec* types I, II, and III) or community settings (SCC*mec* types IV and V) [4] and pulsed-field gel electrophoresis (PFGE) that allows the study of local outbreaks and can be complemented by multilocus sequence typing (MLST) for further comparisons with sequences described in the world and available in databases. The results obtained here can be used for the implementation of interventions that would permit us to reduce the spread of resistant *S. aureus* isolates among elderly people, reducing the risk of infections and complications caused by the pathogen. Furthermore, the results may help support clinical decisions aimed at improving the quality of life of this at-risk population.

We found conditions such as living in an LTCF, male gender, a history of surgeries, and a high Charlson Comorbidity Index (CCI) score to be risk factors associated with *S. aureus* carriage, while MRSA carriage was positively associated with male gender. Small- and medium-sized LTCFs were found to play an important role, with the observation of a high prevalence. Furthermore, the prevalence of MRSA was higher in the oropharynx, a site that is usually neglected. We also report for the first time the identification of ST398 in bedridden individuals and LTCF residents in Brazil.

2. Results

2.1. Prevalence of Colonization with S. aureus and MRSA

Samples collected from 226 individuals were analyzed. The overall prevalence of *S. aureus* carriers was 33.6% ($n = 76$), and that of MRSA carriers was 8% ($n = 18$), identified in at least one sampling site. Regarding the prevalence per site, nasal *S. aureus* carriage was identified in 53 individuals, with exclusive nasal carriage in 33 (14.6%). *S. aureus* was identified in oral samples of 34 individuals, with 17 (7.5%) being exclusive oral carriers. Rectal *S. aureus* was identified in 10 individuals, with exclusive rectal carriage in five (2.2%). In addition, simultaneous nasal and oral carriage was found in 16 (7%) individuals, simultaneous nasal and rectal carriage in four (1.7%), and simultaneous oral and rectal carriage in one (0.4%). Among the 20 MRSA identified, seven originated from nasal samples, eight from oropharyngeal samples, one from a rectal sample, and four simultaneously from nasal and oral samples (Figure 1). It is worth mentioning that nasal methicillin-susceptible *S. aureus* (MSSA) and oral MRSA were identified in one individual, and nasal MRSA and rectal MSSA in another.

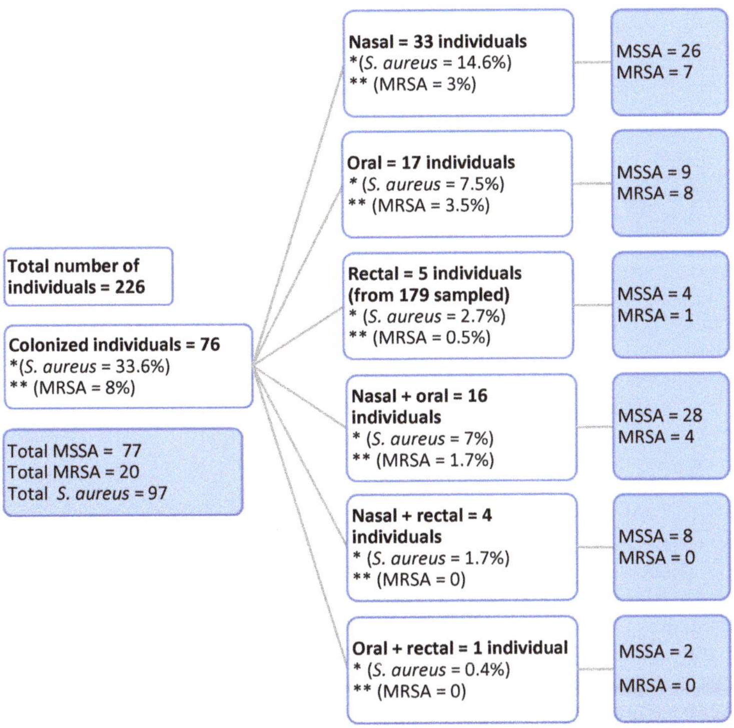

Figure 1. Flow chart of the total number of individuals colonized with *S. aureus* and number of individuals colonized with methicillin-susceptible *S. aureus* (MSSA) and methicillin-resistant *S. aureus* (MRSA) according to the sampling site. Note: Total number of individuals included in the study (226), number of individuals colonized with *S. aureus* (76), and number of colonized individuals according to the sampling site. * Overall prevalence of *S. aureus*. ** Overall prevalence of MRSA.

Among the 226 individuals, 150 were from nine different LTCFs. These facilities vary in size, arbitrarily classified as small (<15 residents), medium-sized (15–49 residents) or large (50 or more residents). Table 1 shows the number of residents per LTCF, which were designated A to I.

Table 1. Prevalence of *S. aureus* and MRSA in long-term care facilities.

Prevalence		LTCF																	
		A (N = 7) Small		B (N = 6) Small		C (N = 12) Small		D (N = 6) Small		E (N = 7) Small		F (N = 18) Medium		G (N = 60) Large		H (N = 16) Medium		I (N = 18) Medium	
		N	%	N	%	N	%	N	%	N	%	N	%	N	%	N	%	N	%
Total	*S. aureus*	6	85.7	3	50.0	7	58.3	2	33.3	3	42.9	5	27.7	20	33.3	8	50.0	3	16.6
	MRSA	1	14.3	1	16.7	0	0	0	0	0	0	0	0	8	13.3	4	25.0	0	0
Nasal	*S. aureus*	4	57.1	1	16.7	1	8.3	2	33.3	0	0	2	11.1	12	20.0	3	18.7	2	11.1
	MRSA	0	0	0	0	0	0	0	0	0	0	0	0	4	6.6	2	12.5	0	0
Oral	*S. aureus*	1	14.3	1	16.7	3	25.0	0	0	1	14.3	0	0	3	5.0	3	18.7	1	5.5
	MRSA	1	14.3	1	16.7	0	0	0	0	0	0	0	0	3	5.0	2	12.5	0	0
Rectal	*S. aureus*	0	0	0	0	0	0	0	0	1	14.3	2	11.1	0	0	0	0	0	0
	MRSA	0	0	0	0	0	0	0	0	0	0	0	0	0	0	0	0	0	0
Nasal + Oral	*S. aureus*	1	14.3	1	16.7	2	16.7	0	0	0	0	1	5.5	3	5.0	2	12.5	0	0
	MRSA	0	0	0	0	0	0	0	0	0	0	0	0	1	1.6	0	0	0	0
Nasal + Rectal	*S. aureus*	0	0	0	0	1	8.3	0	0	0	0	0	0	2	3.3	0	0	0	0
	MRSA	0	0	0	0	0	0	0	0	0	0	0	0	0	0	0	0	0	0
Oral + Rectal	*S. aureus*	0	0	0	0	0	0	0	0	1	14.3	0	0	0	0	0	0	0	0
	MRSA	0	0	0	0	0	0	0	0	0	0	0	0	0	0	0	0	0	0

Note: Prevalence of *S. aureus* and methicillin-resistant *S. aureus* (MRSA) in nine long-term care facilities for the elderly (LTCF), designated A to I.

The prevalence of *S. aureus* in each LTCF was 85.7% (six of the seven in A), 50.0% (three of the six in B), 58.3% (seven of the 12 in C), 33.3% (two of the six in D), 42.9% (three of the seven in E), 27.7% (five of the 18 in F), 33.3% (20 of the 60 in G), 50.0% (eight of the 16 in H), and 16.6% (three of the 18 in I). Residents in only four of the nine facilities were colonized with MRSA, with a prevalence of 14.3% (A), 16.7% (B), 13.3% (G), and 25% (H). Some small facilities had a higher prevalence of *S. aureus* than the other LTCFs.

Twenty (26.3%) of the 76 bedridden patients from whom samples were collected were colonized with *S. aureus*. Of these, four (5.2%) were colonized with MRSA and were mainly from the same neighborhood.

2.2. *In Vitro Antimicrobial Susceptibility Testing*

Analysis of the 97 *S. aureus* isolates from bedridden or institutionalized individuals showed that 11 isolates were resistant to oxacillin and cefoxitin, five were resistant only to oxacillin, and two were resistant only to cefoxitin, corresponding to 18 isolates with phenotypic resistance.

It is important to note that there were isolates that were resistant to oxacillin in vitro and that did not carry the *mecA* gene. In addition, some isolates were phenotypically susceptible to oxacillin and cefoxitin and carried the *mecA* gene. In this study, we classified isolates carrying the *mecA* gene as MRSA, regardless of the phenotypic result observed in the susceptibility tests.

We found no cases of resistance to sulfamethoxazole/trimethoprim, quinupristin/dalfopristin or linezolid, and the vancomycin MIC showed that all isolates were susceptible (Table 2).

Table 2. Antimicrobial susceptibility profile of MSSA and MRSA isolated from bedridden or institutionalized individuals.

S. aureus (*n* = 97)	*mecA* Gene	Oxacillin		Cefoxitin		Linezolid		Q/D		S/T		Vancomycin MIC # (μg/mL)
		R	S	R	S	R	S	R	S	R	S	
MSSA (*n* = 77)	0	3 *	74	0	77	0	77	0	77	0	77	0.19–1.5
MRSA (*n* = 20)	20	13	7 **	13	7 **	0	20	0	20	0	20	0.19–1.5
Total (*n* = 97)	20	16	81	13	84	0	97	0	97	0	97	0.19–1.5

Note: Isolates identified as MSSA and MRSA based on the presence of the *mecA* gene. R: resistant. S: susceptible. Q/D: quinupristin/dalfopristin. S/T: sulfamethoxazole/trimethoprim. MIC: minimum inhibitory concentration. # Range of vancomycin susceptibility obtained for *mecA* gene-negative (MSSA) and -positive (MRSA) isolates. * Isolates resistant to oxacillin that did not carry the *mecA*. ** Isolates susceptible to oxacillin and cefoxitin that carried the *mecA* gene.

2.3. Detection of the mecA Gene and SCCmec Characterization

The *mecA* gene was identified in *S. aureus* isolated from 18 individuals but totaling 20 samples since two individuals carried more than one resistant isolate. Thus, among the 20 resistant isolates, seven originated from nasal samples, eight from the oropharynx, one from a rectal sample, and four from both nasal and oral samples.

Among the 20 *mecA* gene-positive isolates, six carried SCC*mec* type IV (CA-MRSA), nine carried SCC*mec* type II (HA-MRSA), and one carried SCC*mec* type I (HA-MRSA). The remaining isolates could not be typed by the method of Milheiriço et al. [17].

It is important to highlight that all six SCC*mec* type IV found in the study originated from LTCF residents. The nine SCC*mec* type II were identified in three bedridden patients and in six LTCF residents. The only SCC*mec* type I was found in a bedridden patient.

2.4. Risk Factors for MRSA Carriage

The results of univariate and multivariate analysis (logistic regression model) for identifying risk factors associated with *S. aureus* and MRSA carriage are shown in Tables 3 and 4.

For *S. aureus* carriage, a positive association with the time at risk (months of bedriddenness or institutionalization) was only found in univariate analysis ($p = 0.003$). In multivariate analysis, there were positive associations with living in LTCFs (OR = 2.05, 95 %CI = 1.07–3.91, $p = 0.03$), a history of surgeries in the last year (OR = 5.99, 95 %CI = 1.26–28.92, $p = 0.02$) and presence of comorbidities according to the Charlson Comorbidity Index (CCI) score (OR = 1.35, 95 %CI = 1.01–1.92, $p = 0.047$), and a negative association with heart disease (OR = 0.18, 95 %CI = 0.05–0.70, $p = 0.01$). Male gender was positively associated with *S. aureus* carriage in univariate (OR = 2.15, 95 %CI = 1.22–3.79, $p = 0.008$) and multivariate analysis (OR = 2.59, 95 %CI = 1.41–4.76, $p = 0.002$).

Regarding MRSA carriage, univariate (OR = 2.96, 95 %CI = 1.103–7.98, $p = 0.03$) and multivariate (OR = 3.29, 95 %CI = 1.18–9.17, $p = 0.02$) analysis revealed a positive association with male gender.

Table 3. Univariate and multivariate analysis (logistic regression model) of predictors of *S. aureus* carriage.

Risk Factors	Univariate Analysis				Multivariate Analysis	
	S. aureus (*n* = 76)	Negative (*n* = 150)	OR (95 %CI)	*p*	OR (95 %CI)	*p*
Demographic data Male gender	**37 (48.7)**	**48 (30.7)**	**2.15 (1.22–3.79)**	**0.008**	**2.59 (1.41–4.76)**	**0.002**
Age [years], median (quartile)	77.5 (70–84)	80 (70–85)	...	0.41		
Living in a long-term care facility	56 (73.7)	94 (62.7)	1.6 (0.908–3.065)	0.98	**2.05 (1.07–3.91)**	**0.03**
Time at risk * [months], median (quartile)	**36 (12–66)**	**66 (24–66)**	...	**0.003**		

Table 3. *Cont.*

Risk Factors	Univariate Analysis				Multivariate Analysis	
	S. aureus (*n* = 76)	Negative (*n* = 150)	OR (95 %CI)	*p*	OR (95 %CI)	*p*
Comorbidities						
Heart disease	3 (3.9)	17 (11.3)	0.32 (0.01–1.13)	0.07	**0.18 (0.05–0.70)**	**0.01**
Lung disease	5 (6.6)	8 (5.3)	1.25 (0.40–3.96)	0.77		
Kidney disease	4 (5.3)	3 (2.0)	2.72 (0.59–12.48)	0.22		
Liver disease	0 (0.0)	2 (1.3)	0.00 (. . . – . . .)	0.55		
Diabetes mellitus	19 (25.0)	29 (19.3)	1.39 (0.72–2.68)	0.32		
Central nervous system disease	20 (26.3)	33 (22.0)	1.26 (0.66–2.40)	0.46		
Cancer	6 (7.9)	6 (4.0)	2.057 (0.64–6.60)	0.21		
AIDS	0 (0.0)	1 (0.7)	0.00 (. . . – . . .)	1.00		
Pressure ulcer	6 (7.9)	9 (6.0)	1.34 (0.46–3.92)	0.58		
Charlson Comorbidity Index, median (quartile)	1 (1–1)	1 (0–1)	. . .	0.25	**1.35 (1.01–1.92)**	**0.047**
Procedures						
Hospitalization **	14 (18.4)	19 (12.7)	1.55 (0.73–3.30)	0.24		
Surgery **	6 (7.9)	3 (2.0)	4.20 (1.020–17.28)	0.064	**5.99 (1.26–28.92)**	**0.02**
Other invasive procedures **	4 (5.3)	7 (4.7)	1.13 (0.32–4.004)	1.00		
Antimicrobial use **	10 (13.2)	9 (6.0)	2.37 (0.92–6.11)	0.67		

Note: Data are reported as percentages, except when otherwise specified. Significant results are shown in bold. OR: odds ratio. CI: confidence interval. * Time spent in a long-term care facility or bedridden. ** In the last 6 months.

Table 4. Univariate and multivariate analysis (logistic regression model) of predictors of MRSA carriage.

Risk Factors	Univariate Analysis				Multivariate Analysis	
	MRSA (*n* = 18)	Negative (*n* = 208)	OR (95 %CI)	*p*	OR (95 %CI)	*p*
Demographic data						
Male gender	**11 (61.1)**	**72 (34.6)**	**2.96 (1.103–7.98)**	**0.03**	**3.29 (1.18–9.17)**	**0.02**
Age [years], median (quartile)	76 (69.5–83)	77 (60–85)	. . .	0.51		
Living in a long-term care facility	14 (77.8)	136 (65.4)	1.85 (0.58–5.83)	0.28		
Time at risk * [months], median (quartile)	36 (18–67.5)	60 (18–66)		0.61		
Comorbidities						
Heart disease	2 (11.1)	18 (8.7)	1.31 (0.28–6.20)	0.66		
Lung disease	2 (11.1)	11 (5.3)	2.39 (0.45–10.98)	0.27		
Kidney disease	1 (5.6)	6 (2.9)	1.98 (0.22–17.41)	0.44		
Liver disease	0 (0.0)	2 (1.0)	0.00 (. . . – . . .)	1.00		
Diabetes mellitus	1 (5.6)	47 (22.6)	0.20 (0.26–1.55)	0.13		
Central nervous system disease	5 (27.8)	48 (23.1)	1.28 (0.43–3.77)	0.77		
Cancer	1 (5.6)	11 (5.3)	1.053 (0.12–8.65)	1.00		
AIDS	0 (0.0)	1 (0.5)	0.00 (. . . – . . .)	1.00		

Table 4. *Cont.*

Risk Factors	Univariate Analysis				Multivariate Analysis	
	MRSA (*n* = 18)	Negative (*n* = 208)	OR (95 %CI)	*p*	OR (95 %CI)	*p*
Pressure ulcer	3 (16.7)	12 (5.8)	3.26 (0.83–12.85)	0.10		
Charlson Comorbidity Index, median (quartile)	1 (1–1.5)	1 (0–1)	...	0.91		
Procedures						
Hospitalization **	4 (22.2)	29 (13.9)	1.76 (0.54–5.73)	0.30		
Surgery **	1 (5.6)	8 (3.8)	1.47 (0.17–12.46)	0.53		
Other invasive procedures **	1 (5.6)	10 (4.8)	1.16 (0.14–9.65)	1.00		
Antimicrobial use **	2 (11.1)	17 (8.2)	1.40 (0.29–6.62)	0.65		

Note: Data are reported as percentages, except when otherwise specified. Significant results are shown in bold. OR: odds ratio. CI: confidence interval. * Time spent in a long-term care facility or bedridden. ** In the last 6 months.

2.5. Determination of the Clonal Profile of MRSA Isolates by Pulsed-Field Gel Electrophoresis

The 20 *mecA* gene-positive isolates were analyzed by PFGE. Analysis of the dendrogram revealed the presence of clusters with similarity $\geq$ 80% (Figures 2 and 3).

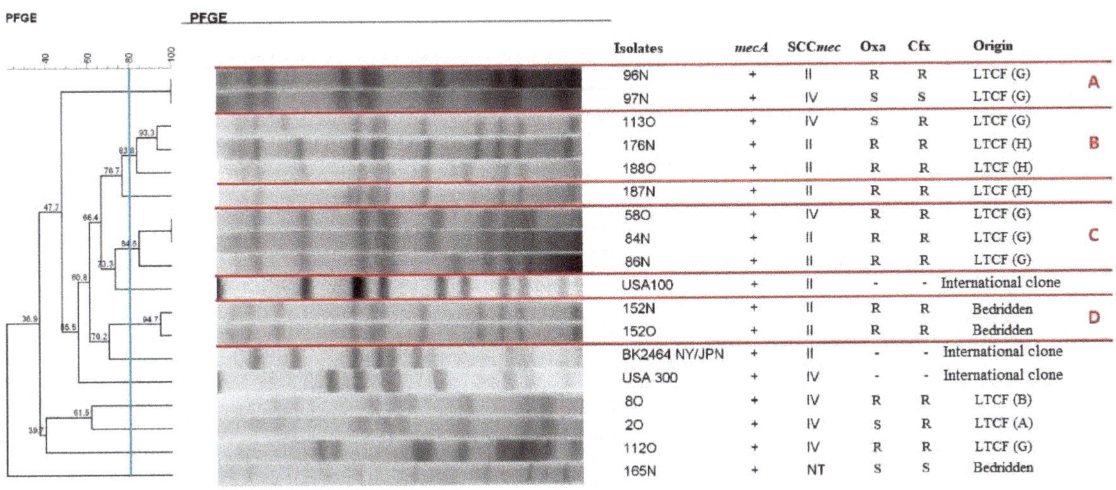

Figure 2. Dendrogram of PFGE-*SmaI* profiles of MRSA isolated from bedridden patients at home or long-term care facility residents generated by Dice analysis/UPGMA (BioNumerics, Applied Maths). Note: N: nasal mucosa. O: oropharyngeal mucosa. NT: not typed. Oxa: oxacillin. Cfx: cefoxitin. S: susceptible. R: resistant. LTCF: long-term care facility. ABCD letters represent clusters, lineages that showed 80% or more similarity.

Figure 2 shows the presence of four MRSA clusters after digestion with *SmaI*. Cluster A comprised two isolates from different individuals (96N and 97N) but from the same LTCF. Cluster B consisted of three isolates from different individuals (113O, 176N, and 188O), one of them living in a different LTCF. Cluster C also comprised three isolates from different individuals (58O, 84N, and 86N), all of them from the same LTCF. Cluster D consisted of two isolates (152N and 152O) from the same bedridden patient.

MRSA that was not digested with *SmaI* were submitted to PFGE typing using *ApaI* (Figure 3). Analysis of the dendrogram revealed the formation of two clusters typed with *ApaI*. Cluster E comprised two isolates (106N and 106O) from different sites of the same institutionalized individuals, while cluster F consisted of MRSA isolates from two individuals (174O and 136O), one isolated from an LTCF resident and the other from a bedridden patient.

It is important to mention that four of the five clusters identified in this study were found in facility G.

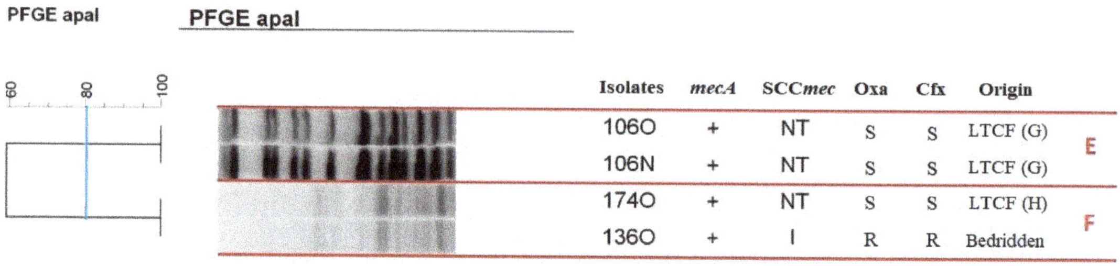

Figure 3. Dendrogram of PFGE-ApaI profiles of MRSA isolated from bedridden patients at home or long-term care facility residents generated by Dice analysis/UPGMA (BioNumerics, Applied Maths). Note: N: nasal mucosa. O: oropharyngeal mucosa. NT: not typed. Oxa: oxacillin. Cfx: cefoxitin. S: susceptible. R: resistant. LTCF: long-term care facility. E and F letter represent clusters, lineages that showed 80% or more similarity.

2.6. Molecular Typing of MRSA by Multilocus Sequence Typing

Based on the diversity found in PFGE and ensuring the choice of representative strains from each cluster identified, nine of the MRSA were selected for MLST typing. Five isolates were ST105, two isolates were ST5, and two were ST398 (Figure 4).

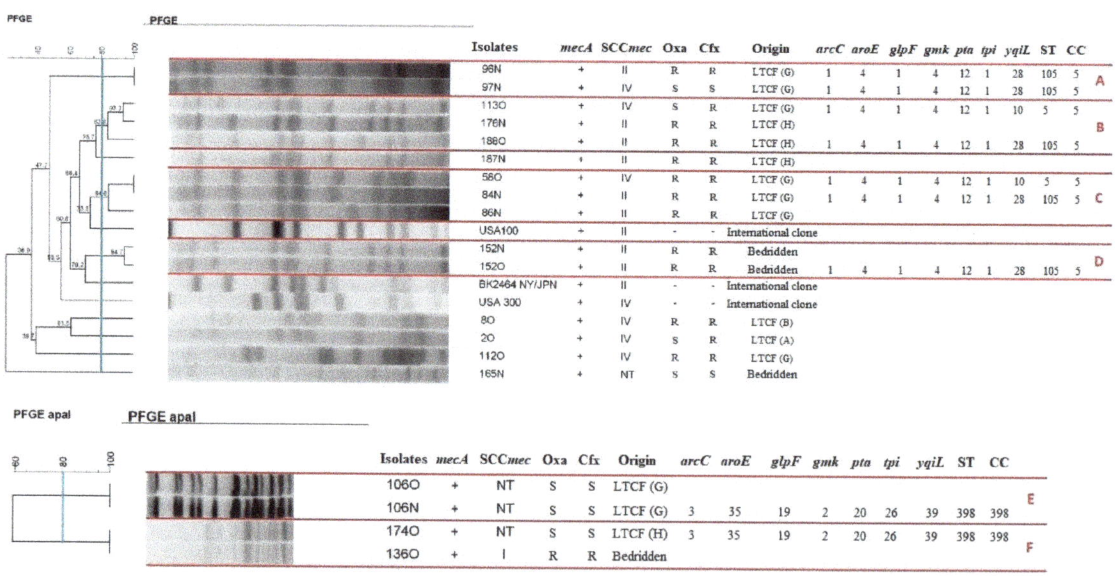

Figure 4. Dendrogram of PFGE-*SmaI* and PFGE-*ApaI* profiles of MRSA isolated from bedridden patients or institutionalized individuals generated by Dice analysis/UPGMA (BioNumerics, Applied Maths) and sequence types (ST) obtained by MLST. Note: Resistant isolates forming clusters >80% similarity after digestion with *SmaI* (clusters A, B, C, D) and *ApaI* (clusters E and F). N: nasal mucosa. O: oropharyngeal mucosa. LTCF: long-term care facility. *arcC*: carbamate kinase. *aroE*: shikimate dehydrogenase. *glpF*: glycerol kinase. *gmk*: guanylate kinase. *pta*: phosphate acetyltransferase. *tpi*: triosephosphate isomerase. *yqiL*: acetyl coenzyme A acetyltransferase. ST: sequence type. CC: clonal complex.

3. Discussion

A multicenter study investigating elderly nursing home residents in France found a prevalence of *S. aureus* and MRSA of 27.6% and 8.7%, respectively [18]. Another multicenter study conducted in Germany identified *S. aureus* as the most prevalent pathogenic agent among nursing home residents, with a prevalence of *S. aureus* of 29.5% and of MRSA of 1.1% [19].

Studying bedridden patients at home and LTCF residents, we found a prevalence of *S. aureus* of 33.6% and of MRSA of 8%. These percentages are similar to those reported in France [18] and Germany [19]. However, the prevalence we found here is higher compared to national data [20]. In a study conducted in a neighboring municipality 94 km away, Silveira et al. [20] observed colonization rates with *S. aureus* and MRSA of 17.7% and 3.7%, respectively, among elderly persons living in nursing homes. A similar prevalence of colonization with *S. aureus* has been reported in the population-based study by Pires et al. [21] among individuals of different ages from the same municipality (prevalence of *S. aureus* of 32.7%); however, our prevalence of MRSA (8%) was higher than that reported by these authors (0.9%).

The prevalence of *S. aureus* and MRSA in nursing homes can vary according to the number of residents. In the present study, the prevalence of MRSA was 13.3% in LTCF G (60 residents) but 25.0% in LTCF H (16 residents). Silveira et al. [20] also observed a higher prevalence of *S. aureus* and MRSA in small- and medium-sized facilities.

Among the bedridden patients at home, 20 (26.3%) of the 76 individuals were colonized with *S. aureus*. Of these, four (5.2%) were colonized with MRSA and were mainly from the same neighborhood, indicating dissemination due to proximity between houses.

Although the nasopharynx is the most consistent site of colonization with *S. aureus* and is indicated as the most appropriate site for swab screening [7], other sites (extranasal) can also be colonized. Recent studies have shown that a substantial number of individuals (7% to 32%) are oropharynx-only carriers of *S. aureus*. These findings suggest that the inclusion of a throat swab in addition to a nasal swab may be important for the success of surveillance programs [22]. Furthermore, eight of the 20 MRSA isolates of the study were only isolated from oral samples and one only from a rectal sample, highlighting the importance of extranasal sites in the epidemiology of this microorganism. These sites are commonly neglected and may contribute to the spread of the pathogen [23]. Almost half (45%) of the MRSA isolates would have been lost if other sites had not been sampled. This fact was also observed by Srinivasan et al. [24], who reported a rate of 28% of MRSA that would be lost if extranasal sites had not been sampled. The presence of MRSA at these sites also indicates a high burden and the risk of dissemination of the pathogen, with the risk of infection being significantly higher in the case of simultaneous colonization of different sites [24].

All SCC*mec* type IV strains were isolated from institutionalized individuals and were considered to be originally community-acquired [4]. SCC*mec* type II, the most prevalent in the present study, was isolated from LTCF residents and from bedridden patients, while type I was found only in one bedridden individual. These findings agree with the study by Silveira et al. [20] that found a higher prevalence of SCC*mec* type II. The authors attributed this fact to the history of hospitalizations since both type II and type I are typical of hospital-associated strains.

It is worth mentioning that individuals who are bedridden at home receive sporadic visits from health agents because of their difficulty in locomotion, a fact that can facilitate the transmission of these microorganisms. This population thus represents a link between the two environments (community and hospital) that directly influences the epidemiological dynamics of *S. aureus* and MRSA [16].

Logistic regression analysis of risk factors for colonization with *S. aureus* revealed a positive association with institutionalization. Elderly institutionalized persons live in a confined environment and often share objects with several residents, a fact that facilitates cross-transmission in these places. In addition, the frequent cognitive impairment of these individuals reduces adherence to basic hygiene measures [13]. A positive association was also observed between *S. aureus* carriage and higher median CCI scores, in agreement with the literature since the presence of a larger number of comorbidities increases the risk of colonization with *S. aureus* [12].

A history of surgeries was also positively associated with *S. aureus* carriage. Surgical site infections can be caused by microorganisms that enter the operative wound either during or after surgery, and *S. aureus* has been described as the most common cause [25]. However, this is not true when we look at the negative association observed with heart disease, which might be explained by competition with other species since 33% to 62.5% of wound infections after heart surgery are caused by coagulase-negative staphylococci [26].

Male gender was positively associated with *S. aureus* carriage and was also the only variable that showed a positive association with MRSA carriage. Studies had previously reported a higher risk of MRSA transmission among male residents of LTCFs when compared to women, probably because the former have more risk factors. In this regard, more frequent damage to the skin barrier may represent a confounder for the risk factor 'male gender.' Another explanation would be biased selection in which the analyses included more men instead of case-matched controls [27,28]. Colonization may even be related to hormonal differences [29].

PFGE typing of MRSA isolated from bedridden or institutionalized individuals revealed the formation of six clusters, four of them comprising MRSA isolates from LTCF G, which had the largest number of residents as well as the largest number of MRSA isolates (9 [45%] of the 20 MRSA found in the study). Studies have shown a higher risk of colonization with MRSA across the nursing team [30], and LTCF G had a larger group of professionals than the other institutions in the study. The PFGE results also showed the formation of a cluster consisting of MRSA from LTCF G and MRSA from another medium-sized facility, indicating the spread of MRSA between different facilities. Although we cannot confirm the role of health assistants and their influence on the dissemination between the facilities since we did not investigate this issue in our study, it is important to note that different institutions tend to be attended by the same health units with a visit from the nursing team that can act as vectors. MRSA typing also revealed a similarity between one MRSA strain isolated from a bedridden patient and MRSA isolated from the medium-sized LTCF. The dissemination of persistent clones in the community requires attention since it puts the population at increased risk of infection. The different reservoirs in the community facilitate the transmission of endemic strains to households [31]. Silveira et al. [20] also found evidence of transmission between LTCFs for three clusters identified in their study.

Strain ST398 is a new livestock-associated MRSA clonal lineage that can infect or colonize humans even in the absence of exposure to livestock animals [32]. A Dutch study found that ST398 was able to spread in a nursing home, affecting seven residents and four employees [33]. Here we identified ST398 in a bedridden individual and in two residents of different LTCFs (G and H). Our study is the first to report the identification of ST398 in bedridden or institutionalized individuals in Brazil.

The data obtained may contribute to what is already known about the epidemiology of *S. aureus* and MRSA and to the identification of risk factors associated with the carriage of these microorganisms in the population studied. In conclusion, we believe that interventions are necessary in nursing homes in order to improve the quality of life and to help control the spread of these pathogens within the community. We also strongly encourage the inclusion of extranasal sites in MRSA screening.

4. Materials and Methods

4.1. Study Design

This cross-sectional study was conducted in Botucatu, SP, Brazil, where 188 LTCF residents and 222 bedridden patients were registered with the Health Department of the city. The sample size was calculated using the formula described in Appendix A, which suggested an n of 173 individuals.

The individuals were contacted during home visits and visits to the LTCF and were invited to participate in the study. The elderly persons agreed to participate by signing the free informed consent form. In the case of cognitive deficit, consent was obtained from the legal representative or, in his/her absence, from the nursing home. A questionnaire (Appendix B) containing the following data was also applied: demographic data (gender and age), time of institutionalization, clinical data (comorbidities), use of invasive devices, recent hospitalizations (last 6 months), current or recent infectious diseases, and use of antimicrobial agents (last 6 months). These data were obtained through interviews with the participants and/or their legal representatives.

4.2. Inclusion and Exclusion Criteria

All individuals who agreed to participate in the study were included. In the case of inability to understand, the individual was included after consent was obtained from the legal representative. Individuals institutionalized or bedridden for less than 30 days were excluded.

4.3. Sample Collection

Samples were collected from the nasal vestibule, oropharynx and rectum of 226 individuals (150 residents of nine LTCFs and 76 bedridden individuals at home) in the city of Botucatu, SP, Brazil, with a sterile swab specific for each site. Because of the refusal of 47 individuals, only 179 rectal swabs were collected. There were no refusals of nasal or oral swab collection.

Nasal samples were collected by moistening the swab in 0.9% saline (sterile technique) and introducing it into both nostrils until the maximum depth that could be tolerated by the participant. The rod was rotated, gently pressing the end against the mucosa. For oropharyngeal sampling, the swab was gently pressed and rotated over the tonsils and behind the uvula (posterior pharynx), avoiding touching the tongue, buccal mucosa, and uvula. For the collection of rectal samples, the tip of the swab was passed approximately 2 cm from the anal sphincter, rotating it carefully to collect a sample from the anal crypts and ensuring that there was fecal staining on the cotton after removal of the swab. After collection, the swabs were transported in Stuart's medium to the Laboratory of Microbiology, Department of Microbiology and Immunology, Botucatu Institute of Biosciences.

4.4. Phenotypic Identification of S. aureus

The samples collected from the three sites were seeded onto Petri dishes containing Baird Parker agar, a selective medium for *Staphylococcus*. After incubation for 48 h at 37 °C, the colonies growing on the agar were submitted to Gram staining for assessing purity, observation of morphology, and specific staining. After confirmation of these features, the tube catalase and coagulase tests were performed according to Koneman et al. [34], as well as additional biochemical tests (maltose, trehalose, and mannitol fermentation).

4.5. Genotypic Identification of S. aureus

DNA was extracted using the Illustra Kit (GE Healthcare, Little Chalfont, Buckinghamshire, United Kingdom). After extraction, PCR was performed for amplification of the *Sa442* DNA fragments, which is specific for *S. aureus*, following the protocol described by Martineau et al. [35]. The following primers that amplify a 241-bp fragment were used: *Sa442*-1 (5′-AAT CTT TGT CGG TAC ACG ATA TTC TTC ACG-3′) and *Sa442*-2 (5′-CGT AAT GAG ATT TCA GTA GAT AAT ACA ACA-3′).

4.6. Antimicrobial Susceptibility Tests

All isolates were submitted to antimicrobial susceptibility testing by the disk diffusion method according to the criteria recommended by the Clinical Laboratory Standards Institute (CLSI) [36]. Cultures in BHI broth previously incubated for 18–24 h and adjusted with saline to a 0.5 McFarland turbidity standard were used for the preparation of the inoculum. The following drugs were tested: oxacillin (1 μg), cefoxitin (30 μg), linezolid (30 μg), quinupristin/dalfopristin (15 μg), and sulfamethoxazole/trimethoprim (25 μg). After density adjustment, the inoculum was seeded with a sterile swab on Mueller-Hinton agar, and the drug-impregnated disks were placed on the agar surface. The plates were incubated for 24 h at 35 °C. Antimicrobial activity was evaluated based on the diameter of the inhibition halo, which was interpreted according to the CLSI criteria. The *S. aureus* ATCC 25923 reference strain was used as a control during the test.

4.7. Determination of Minimum Inhibitory Concentration (MIC)

The vancomycin MIC was determined by the E-test. This quantitative method uses inert and transparent plastic strips (60 mm long and 5.5 mm wide) that carry a concentration gradient of the stabilized antimicrobial agent. The results were analyzed following the definitions established by the CLSI [36].

4.8. Molecular Detection of the mecA Gene and Characterization of SCCmec

The PCR assays for the detection of the *mecA* gene (methicillin resistance gene) were performed following the parameters described by Murakami et al. [37]. The following primers that amplify a 533-bp fragment were used: *mecA*1 (5′-AAA ATC GAT GGT AAA GGT TGG C-3′) and *mecA*2 (5′-AGT TCT GCA GTA CCG GAT TTG C-3′). International reference strains were included as positive (*S. aureus* ATCC 33591) and negative controls (*S. aureus* ATCC 25923) in all reactions. The efficiency of the amplifications was monitored by electrophoresis of the reaction on SYBR Safe-stained agarose gel (2%).

SCC*mec* typing was performed by multiplex PCR as described by Oliveira and de Lencastre [38] and updated by Milheiriço et al. [17]. The following reference strains were used: COL for SCC*mec* type I; N315 for SCC*mec* type IA; PER34 for SCC*mec* type II; AN546 for SCC*mec* type III; HU25 for SCC*mec* type IIIA, and MW2 for SCC*mec* type IV.

4.9. Pulsed-Field Gel Electrophoresis (PFGE)

All *mecA* gene-positive isolates obtained in this study were submitted to molecular typing by PFGE, following the modified protocol of McDougal et al. [39]. The MRSA isolates were cultured in BHI broth for 24 h. Next, 400 μL of the sample was added to a microtube and centrifuged at 12,000 rpm for 50 s. The supernatant was discarded, and 300 μL TE solution (10 mM Tris, 1 mM EDTA [pH 8.0]) was added. The samples were left in a water bath at 37 °C for 10 min. After vortexing, 5 μL lysostaphin (1 mg/mL in 20 mM sodium acetate [pH 4.5]) and 300 μL low-melt agarose were added. Agarose plugs of the samples were then prepared. After solidification, the plugs were transferred to a 24-well plate containing 2 mL EC solution (6 mM Tris-HCl, 1 M NaCl, 100 mM EDTA, 0.5% Brij-58, 0.2% sodium deoxycholate, 0.5% laurylsarcosine sodium) and incubated for at least 4 h at 37 °C. After this period, the EC solution was removed, and the plugs were washed four times (intervals of 30 min) with 2 mL TE at room temperature.

The *SmaI* enzyme (Fast Digest *SmaI*, MBI Fermentas Inc. Hamilton, Ontario, Canada) was used for genomic DNA restriction. Electrophoresis on 1% agarose gel prepared with 0.5 M TBE (Pulsed Field Certified Agarose, BioRad Laboratories, Hercules, CA, USA) was carried out in a CHEF-DR III System (BioRad Laboratories, Hercules, CA, USA) under the following conditions: pulse time of 5–40 s for 21 h; linear ramp; 6 V/cm; angle of 120°; 14 °C; 0.5 M TBE as running buffer. The Lambda Ladder PFG (New England BioLabs, Ipswich, Massachusetts, EUA) was used as a molecular marker. The gel was stained with GelRed (10,000× in water; Biotium, Fremont, CA, USA) for 1 h and photographed under UV transillumination.

The BioNumerics software (version 7.6; Applied Maths, Sint-Martens-Latem, Belgium) was used for similarity analysis. The dendrogram was constructed by the UPGMA method (Unweighted Pair Group Method with Arithmetic Mean), adopting a band position tolerance of 1.2% and optimization of 1%. A dice similarity coefficient ≥ 80% was chosen for the definition of clusters.

The *ApaI* restriction enzyme was used for MRSA isolates that could not be typed after digestion with *SmaI*.

4.10. Multilocus Sequence Typing (MLST)

MLST was performed as described by Enright et al. [40]. Each primer pair amplifies an internal fragment of the housekeeping genes (about 500 bp). The following genes were used: carbamate kinase (*arcC*), shikimate dehydrogenase (*aroE*), glycerol kinase (*glpF*), guanylate kinase (*gmk*), phosphate acetyltransferase (*pta*), triosephosphate isomerase (*tpi*), and acetyl coenzyme A acetyltransferase (*yqiL*). The products were purified using the Real Biotech Corp (RBC) HiYield™ Gel/PCR Fragments Extraction Kit. The reactions were carried out in an ABI3500 8-capillary sequencer (50 cm) using POP7 (Applied Biosystems, Waltham, Massachusetts, USA) as polymer. The sequences (electropherograms) were visualized using the BioNumerics program (version 7.6; Applied Maths, Sint-Martens-Latem, Belgium). The sequences were analyzed and compared via an online database (https://pubmlst.org) (accessed on 29 August 2020).

4.11. Statistical Analysis

The study design is cross-sectional, and the presence of *S. aureus* or MRSA was defined as the outcome. For the identification of risk factors, univariate analysis was first performed. Dichotomous variables were analyzed using the chi-squared test or Fisher's exact test when appropriate. Numerical variables were compared by the Mann-Whitney U test. We then tested confounding in multivariate logistic regression models using a stepwise forward selection strategy, with $p < 0.1$ being adopted as a criterion for entry and continuation of the variables in the models. The data were stored in EPI INFO 7 (Centers for Disease Control and Prevention, Atlanta, GA, USA), and all analyses were performed using SPSS 20 (IBM, Armonk, NY, USA).

Author Contributions: Carried out the experiments, analyzed the data and drafted the manuscript, L.P.S.; conceived the study, participated in study design, analyzed the data, C.M.C.B.F.; contributed to the laboratory experiments, N.B.T., L.T.P.S., C.D.d.A.; conceived the study, participated in its design and coordination and revised the manuscript, M.d.L.R.d.S.d.C. All authors have read and agreed to the published version of the manuscript.

Funding: This study was funded by the São Paulo State Research Foundation (FAPESP—Grant 2017/21396-0), the National Council for Scientific and Technological Development (CNPq—Grant 303603/2020-8) and Coordination for Improvement of Higher Education Personnel (CAPES—Grant 88882.183592/2018-01).

Institutional Review Board Statement: The present study was approved by the Research Ethics Committee of the Botucatu Medical School, São Paulo State, Brazil (Approval number 2.447.581).

Informed Consent Statement: Informed consent was obtained from all subjects involved in the study.

Data Availability Statement: The data presented in this study are contained within the article.

Acknowledgments: We thank the São Paulo State Research Foundation (FAPESP—Grant 2017/21396-0 and Grant 2020/15118-0) and the Coordination for Improvement of Higher Education Personnel (CAPES—Grant 88882.183592/2018-01).

Conflicts of Interest: The authors declare no conflict of interest.

Appendix A

Sample size formula

A representative sample was selected based on the following parameters:

- Population size (finite population correlation factor or FCP) (N): 350;
- Hypothetical % frequency of the outcome factor in the population (p): 33% $\pm$ 5;
- Confidence limits as % of 100 (absolute $\pm$%) (d): 5%;
- Design effect (DEFF): 1;

- Equation: $n = [DEFF * Np(1 - p)]/[(d2/Z21 - \alpha/2 * (N - 1) + p * (1 - p)]$;
- Sample size (95% confidence interval): 173.

Appendix B Questionnaire

Name: ______________________________ Gender: _____ Age: ____

Nursing home (Y/N): ______________________________

Time of institutionalization (months): _____ Time of bedriddenness (months): _____

Comorbidities/Charlson Comorbidity Index

1 ( ) AMI ( ) CHF ( ) Peripheral vascular disease
( ) Dementia ( ) COPD ( ) Connective tissue disease
( ) Peptic ulcer ( ) Mild liver disease
( ) Cerebrovascular disease ( ) Diabetes

2 ( ) Hemiplegia ( ) Moderate/severe kidney disease
( ) Malignant neoplasm ( ) Leukemia ( ) Lymphoma
( ) Diabetes with organ damage

3 ( ) Moderate/severe liver disease

4 ( ) AIDS ( ) Solid metastatic tumor

Charlson Comorbidity Index: ______

Other comorbidities: Senile dementia? (Y/N): ____

____

____

____

Karnofsky: ______

Hospitalizations in the last year:

Hospital	Admission Date	Discharge Date	Reason

Use of antimicrobials in the last year:

Antimicrobial	Start Date	End Date	Reason

Surgeries and invasive procedures in the last year:

Procedure	Date	Reason

References

1. Chambers, H. The Changing Epidemiology of *Staphylococcus aureus*? *Emerg. Infect. Dis.* **2001**, *7*, 178–182. [CrossRef] [PubMed]
2. Klein, E.; Sun, L.; Smith, D.; Laxminarayan, R. The Changing Epidemiology of Methicillin-Resistant *Staphylococcus aureus* in the United States: A National Observational Study. *Am. J. Epidemiology* **2013**, *177*, 666–674. [CrossRef]
3. Nimmo, G.R.; Bergh, H.; Nakos, J.; Whiley, D.; Marquess, J.; Huygens, F.; Paterson, D. Replacement of healthcare-associated MRSA by community-associated MRSA in Queensland: Confirmation by genotyping. *J. Infect.* **2013**, *67*, 439–447. [CrossRef] [PubMed]
4. Otto, M. Community-associated MRSA: What makes them special? *Int. J. Med. Microbiol.* **2013**, *303*, 324–330. [CrossRef] [PubMed]
5. Cataldo, M.A.; Taglietti, F.; Petrosillo, N. Methicillin-Resistant *Staphylococcus aureus*: A Community Health Threat. *Postgrad. Med.* **2010**, *122*, 16–23. [CrossRef]
6. Braga, E.D.V.; Aguiar-Alves, F.; Freitas, M.D.F.N.D.; De E Silva, M.O.; Correa, T.V.; E Snyder, R.; De Araújo, V.A.; Marlow, M.A.; Riley, L.W.; Setúbal, S.; et al. High prevalence of Staphylococcus aureus and methicillin-resistant *S. aureus colonization* among healthy children attending public daycare centers in informal settlements in a large urban center in Brazil. *BMC Infect. Dis.* **2014**, *14*, 1–10. [CrossRef]
7. Lo, W.-T.; Wang, C.-C.; Lin, W.-J.; Wang, S.-R.; Teng, C.-S.; Huang, C.-F.; Chen, S.-J. Changes in the Nasal Colonization with Methicillin-Resistant *Staphylococcus aureus* in Children: 2004-2009. *PLoS ONE* **2010**, *5*, e15791. [CrossRef]
8. Tong, S.Y.C.; Chen, L.F.; Fowler, V.G. Colonization, pathogenicity, host susceptibility, and therapeutics for *Staphylococcus aureus*: What is the clinical relevance? *Semin. Immunopathol.* **2011**, *34*, 185–200. [CrossRef]
9. Safdar, N.; Bradley, E. The Risk of Infection after Nasal Colonization with *Staphylococcus aureus*. *Am. J. Med.* **2008**, *121*, 310–315. [CrossRef]
10. Rodrigues, M.V.P.; Fortaleza, C.M.C.B.; Souza, C.S.M.; Teixeira, N.B.; Cunha, M.D.L.R.D.S.D. Genetic Determinants of Methicillin Resistance and Virulence among *Staphylococcus aureus* Isolates Recovered from Clinical and Surveillance Cultures in a Brazilian Teaching Hospital. *ISRN Microbiol.* **2012**, *2012*, 975143. [CrossRef]
11. Rebelo, M.; Pereira, B.; Lima, J.; Decq-Mota, J.; Vieira, J.D.; Costa, J.N. Predictors of in-hospital mortality in elderly patients with bacteraemia admitted to an Internal Medicine ward. *Int. Arch. Med.* **2011**, *4*, 33. [CrossRef]
12. Bierowiec, K.; Płoneczka-Janeczko, K.; Rypuła, K. Is the Colonisation of *Staphylococcus aureus* in Pets Associated with Their Close Contact with Owners? *PLoS ONE* **2016**, *11*, e0156052. [CrossRef]
13. Aschbacher, R.; Pagani, E.; Confalonieri, M.; Farina, C.; Fazii, P.; Luzzaro, F.; Montanera, P.G.; Piazza, A.; Pagani, L. Review on colonization of residents and staff in Italian long-term care facilities by multidrug-resistant bacteria compared with other European countries. *Antimicrob. Resist. Infect. Control* **2016**, *5*, 33. [CrossRef] [PubMed]
14. Hughes, C.; Smith, M.; Tunney, M. Infection control strategies for preventing the transmission of meticillin-resistant *Staphylococcus aureus* (MRSA) in nursing homes for older people. *Cochrane Database Syst. Rev.* **2008**, *1*, CD006354. [CrossRef]
15. Jans, B.; Schoevaerdts, D.; Huang, T.-D.; Berhin, C.; Latour, K.; Bogaerts, P.; Nonhoff, C.; Denis, O.; Catry, B.; Glupczynski, Y. Epidemiology of Multidrug-Resistant Microorganisms among Nursing Home Residents in Belgium. *PLoS ONE* **2013**, *8*, e64908. [CrossRef]
16. Lee, B.Y.; Bartsch, S.M.; Wong, K.F.; Singh, A.; Avery, T.R.; Kim, D.S.; Brown, S.; Murphy, C.R.; Yilmaz, S.L.; Potter, M.A.; et al. The Importance of Nursing Homes in the Spread of Methicillin-resistant *Staphylococcus aureus* (MRSA) Among Hospitals. *Med. Care* **2013**, *51*, 205–215. [CrossRef]
17. Milheiriço, C.; Oliveira, D.C.; de Lencastre, H. Update to the Multiplex PCR Strategy for Assignment of *mec* Element Types in *Staphylococcus aureus*. *Antimicrob. Agents Chemother.* **2007**, *51*, 3374–3377. [CrossRef]
18. Rondeau, C.; Chevet, G.; Blanc, D.; Gbaguidi-Haore, H.; Decalonne, M.; Dos Santos, S.; Quentin, R.; Van Der Mee-Marquet, N. Current Molecular Epidemiology of Methicillin-Resistant *Staphylococcus aureus* in Elderly French People: Troublesome Clones on the Horizon. *Front. Microbiol.* **2016**, *7*, 31. [CrossRef]
19. Kwetkat, A.; Pfister, W.; Pansow, D.; Pletz, M.W.; Sieber, C.C.; Hoyer, H. Naso- and oropharyngeal bacterial carriage in nursing home residents: Impact of multimorbidity and functional impairment. *PLoS ONE* **2018**, *13*, e0190716. [CrossRef]
20. Da Silveira, M.; Cunha, M.D.L.R.D.S.D.; De Souza, C.S.M.; Correa, A.A.F.; Fortaleza, C.M.C.B. Nasal colonization with methicillin-resistant *Staphylococcus aureus* among elderly living in nursing homes in Brazil: Risk factors and molecular epidemiology. *Ann. Clin. Microbiol. Antimicrob.* **2018**, *17*, 18. [CrossRef]
21. Pires, F.V.; Cunha, M.D.L.R.D.S.D.; Abraao, L.M.; Martins, P.Y.F.; Camargo, C.; Fortaleza, C.M.C.B. Nasal Carriage of *Staphylococcus aureus* in Botucatu, Brazil: A Population-Based Survey. *PLoS ONE* **2014**, *9*, e92537. [CrossRef]

22. Smith, T.C.; Forshey, B.M.; Hanson, B.M.; Wardyn, S.E.; Moritz, E.D. Molecular and epidemiologic predictors of *Staphylococcus aureus* colonization site in a population with limited nosocomial exposure. *Am. J. Infect. Control* **2012**, *40*, 992–996. [CrossRef] [PubMed]
23. Hamdan-Partida, A.; Sainz-Espuñes, T.; Bustos-Martínez, J. Characterization and Persistence of *Staphylococcus aureus* Strains Isolated from the Anterior Nares and Throats of Healthy Carriers in a Mexican Community. *J. Clin. Microbiol.* **2010**, *48*, 1701–1705. [CrossRef]
24. Srinivasan, A.; Seifried, S.E.; Zhu, L.; Srivastava, D.K.; Bs, R.P.; Shenep, J.L.; Bankowski, M.J.; Hayden, R.T. Increasing prevalence of nasal and rectal colonization with methicillin-resistant Staphylococcus aureus in children with cancer. *Pediatr. Blood Cancer* **2010**, *55*, 1317–1322. [CrossRef]
25. Juyal, D.; Pal, S.; Sayana, A.; Joshi, A. *Staphylococcus aureus*: A predominant cause of surgical site infections in a rural healthcare setup of Uttarakhand. *J. Fam. Med. Prim. Care* **2019**, *8*, 3600–3606. [CrossRef]
26. Bitkover, C.Y.; Marcusson, E.; Ransjö, U. Spread of coagulase-negative staphylococci during cardiac operations in a modern operating room. *Ann. Thorac. Surg.* **2000**, *69*, 1110–1115. [CrossRef]
27. Nillius, D.; von Müller, L.; Wagenpfeil, S.; Klein, R.; Herrmann, M. Methicillin-Resistant *Staphylococcus aureus* in Saarland, Germany: The Long-Term Care Facility Study. *PLoS ONE* **2016**, *11*, e0153030. [CrossRef] [PubMed]
28. Couderc, C.; Jolivet, S.; Thiébaut, A.C.M.; Ligier, C.; Remy, L.; Alvarez, A.-S.; Lawrence, C.; Salomon, J.; Herrmann, J.-L.; Guillemot, D.; et al. Fluoroquinolone Use Is a Risk Factor for Methicillin-Resistant *Staphylococcus aureus* Acquisition in Long-term Care Facilities: A Nested Case-Case-Control Study. *Clin. Infect. Dis.* **2014**, *59*, 206–215. [CrossRef]
29. Nowak, J.E.; Borkowska, B.A.; Pawlowski, B.Z. Sex differences in the risk factors for *Staphylococcus aureus* throat carriage. *Am. J. Infect. Control* **2016**, *45*, 29–33. [CrossRef]
30. Dulon, M.; Peters, C.; Schablon, A.; Nienhaus, A. MRSA carriage among healthcare workers in non-outbreak settings in Europe and the United States: A systematic review. *BMC Infect. Dis.* **2014**, *14*, 363. [CrossRef]
31. Knox, J.; Uhlemann, A.-C.; Lowy, F.D. *Staphylococcus aureus* infections: Transmission within households and the community. *Trends Microbiol.* **2015**, *23*, 437–444. [CrossRef]
32. Camoez, M.; Sierra, J.M.; Pujol, M.; Hornero, A.; Martín, R.; Domínguez, M.A. Prevalence and Molecular Characterization of Methicillin-Resistant *Staphylococcus aureus* ST398 Resistant to Tetracycline at a Spanish Hospital over 12 Years. *PLoS ONE* **2013**, *8*, e72828. [CrossRef]
33. Verkade, E.; Bosch, T.; Hendriks, Y.; Kluytmans, J. Outbreak of Methicillin-Resistant *Staphylococcus aureus* ST398 in a Dutch Nursing Home. *Infect. Control Hosp. Epidemiol.* **2012**, *33*, 624–626. [CrossRef]
34. Konemman, E.V.; Allen, S.D.; Sowell, V.R.; Sommer, H.M. Introdução à Microbiologia Médica. In *Diagnóstico Microbiológico: Texto e Atlas Colorido*, 5th ed.; Medsi: Rio de Janeiro, Brazil, 2001.
35. Martineau, F.; Picard, F.J.; Roy, P.H.; Ouellette, M.; Bergeron, M.G. Species-Specific and Ubiquitous-DNA-Based Assays for Rapid Identification of *Staphylococcus aureus*. *J. Clin. Microbiol.* **1998**, *36*, 618–623. [CrossRef]
36. CLSI. *M100S Performance Standards for Antimicrobial Susceptibility Testing*, 26th ed.; Clinical and Laboratory Standards Institute: Wayne, PA, USA, 2016.
37. Murakami, K.; Minamide, W.; Wada, K.; Nakamura, E.; Teraoka, H.; Watanabe, S. Identification of methicillin-resistant strains of staphylococci by polymerase chain reaction. *J. Clin. Microbiol.* **1991**, *29*, 2240–2244. [CrossRef]
38. Oliveira, D.C.; de Lencastre, H. Multiplex PCR Strategy for Rapid Identification of Structural Types and Variants of the *mec* Element in Methicillin-Resistant *Staphylococcus aureus*. *Antimicrob. Agents Chemother.* **2002**, *46*, 2155–2161. [CrossRef]
39. McDougal, L.K.; Steward, C.D.; Killgore, G.E.; Chaitram, J.M.; McAllister, S.K.; Tenover, F.C. Pulsed-Field Gel Electrophoresis Typing of Oxacillin-Resistant *Staphylococcus aureus* Isolates from the United States: Establishing a National Database. *J. Clin. Microbiol.* **2003**, *41*, 5113–5120. [CrossRef]
40. Enright, M.C.; Day, N.P.J.; Davies, C.E.; Peacock, S.J.; Spratt, B.G. Multilocus Sequence Typing for Characterization of Methicillin-Resistant and Methicillin-Susceptible Clones of *Staphylococcus aureus*. *J. Clin. Microbiol.* **2000**, *38*, 1008–1015. [CrossRef]

antibiotics

MDPI

Article

Phenotypic and Genotypic Characterization of Macrolide, Lincosamide and Streptogramin B Resistance among Clinical Methicillin-Resistant *Staphylococcus aureus* Isolates in Chile

Mario Quezada-Aguiluz [1,2,3,4], Alejandro Aguayo-Reyes [1,2,5,6], Cinthia Carrasco [1], Daniela Mejías [1], Pamela Saavedra [1], Sergio Mella-Montecinos [2,5,6], Andrés Opazo-Capurro [1,3,*], Helia Bello-Toledo [1,3], José M. Munita [3,7], Juan C. Hormazábal [8] and Gerardo González-Rocha [1,3,*]

1 Laboratorio de Investigación en Agentes Antibacterianos, Departamento de Microbiología, Facultad de Ciencias Biológicas, Universidad de Concepción, Concepción 4070386, Chile; marioquezada@udec.cl (M.Q.-A.); alejandroaguayo@udec.cl (A.A.-R.); cinthiacarrasco@udec.cl (C.C.); dmejias@udec.cl (D.M.); pame.eudec@gmail.com (P.S.); hbello@udec.cl (H.B.-T.)

2 Departamento de Medicina Interna, Facultad de Medicina, Universidad de Concepción, Concepción 4070386, Chile; pignatio@outlook.com

3 Millennium Initiative for Collaborative Research on Bacterial Resistance (MICROB-R), Santiago 3580000, Chile; munita.jm@gmail.com

4 Centro Regional de Telemedicina y Telesalud del Biobío (CRT Biobío), Concepción 4030000, Chile

5 Unidad de Medicina Interna, Hospital Traumatológico de Concepción, Concepción 4030000, Chile

6 Unidad de Infectología, Hospital Regional "Dr. Guillermo Grant B.", Concepción 4030000, Chile

7 Genomics and Resistant Microbes (GeRM) Group, Facultad de Medicina, Clínica Alemana Universidad del Desarrollo, Santiago 7550000, Chile

8 Subdepartamento de Enfermedades Infecciosas, Instituto de Salud Pública de Chile, Santiago 7780050, Chile; jchormazabal@ispch.cl

* Correspondence: andopazo@udec.cl (A.O.-C.); ggonzal@udec.cl (G.G.-R.)

Abstract: Macrolides, lincosamides, and type B streptogramins (MLS_B) are important therapeutic options to treat methicillin-resistant *Staphylococcus aureus* (MRSA) infections; however, resistance to these antibiotics has been emerging. In Chile, data on the MLS_B resistance phenotypes are scarce in both community-(CA) and hospital-acquired (HA) MRSA isolates. Antimicrobial susceptibility to MLS_B was determined for sixty-eight non-repetitive isolates of each HA-(32) and CA-MRSA (36). Detection of SCC*mec* elements, *ermA*, *ermB*, *ermC*, and *msrA* genes was performed by PCR. The predominant clones were SCC*mec* I-ST5 (HA-MRSA) and type IVc-ST8 (CA-MRSA). Most of the HA-MRSA isolates (97%) showed resistance to clindamycin, erythromycin, azithromycin, and clarithromycin. Among CA-MRSA isolates, 28% were resistant to erythromycin, azithromycin, and 25% to clarithromycin. All isolates were susceptible to linezolid, vancomycin, daptomycin and trimethoprim/sulfamethoxazole, and over 97% to rifampicin. The *ermA* gene was amplified in 88% of HA-MRSA and 17% of CA-MRSA isolates ($p < 0.001$). The *ermC* gene was detected in 6% of HA-SARM and none of CA-SARM isolates, whereas the *msrA* gene was only amplified in 22% of CA-MRSA ($p < 0.005$). Our results demonstrate the prevalence of the cMLSB resistance phenotype in all HA-MRSA isolates in Chile, with the *ermA* being the predominant gene identified among these isolates.

Keywords: MRSA; MLS_B phenotype; antibiotic-resistant

1. Introduction

Methicillin-resistant *Staphylococcus aureus* (MRSA) is an important pathogen involved in both human and animal infections [1,2]. Although MRSA was initially described as producing healthcare-associated infections (HA-MRSA), the appearance of community-associated MRSA infections (CA-MRSA) has been documented since the 1990s [3]. MRSA has shown a remarkable ability to develop resistance to a myriad of antibiotics, as well as to different disinfectants and heavy metals [4]. Vancomycin (VAN), a member of the glycopeptides, has been used as an important option to treat MRSA infections [5]. However, the risk of dissemination of vancomycin-resistant or non-fully susceptible strains suggests that this antibiotic should be used sparingly [6]. For this reason, macrolides (erythromycin [ERY]), lincosamides (clindamycin [CLI]), and streptogramins B (MLS_B) have emerged as important therapeutic options to tackle CA-MRSA infections [7,8]. However, the increased use of these antimicrobials has favored the emergence of resistance to these drugs [9–11]. To date, there are three main MLS_B resistance mechanisms described: i) changes in the ribosomal target site, which confers cross-resistance to the entire MLS_B group [12]. This mechanism is conferred by ribosomal mutations or methylation of the 23S rRNA target site, which are mediated by the *erm* genes (mainly *erm*A, *erm*B, and *erm*C) [13,14]. Another mechanism corresponds to ii) an efflux-pump encoded by *msrA*, which can drive out 14- and 15-membered macrolides and streptogramin B, producing the MS_B phenotype [15]. Finally, another mechanism iii) relies on drug inactivation and it only confers resistance to lincosamides due to an enzyme encoded by the *lnu* gene [11].

Significantly, the MLS_B phenotype can be either constitutive ($cMLS_B$) or inducible ($iMLS_B$) [9]. Specifically, CLI, which is the MLS_B agent used for the treatment of *S. aureus* infections, is a weak MLS_B-resistance inducer and may lead to treatment failure due to false susceptibility results displayed in in vitro antimicrobial susceptibility tests [16]. Therefore, it is necessary to perform the CLI susceptibility test in the presence of a strong inducer, such as ERY [12]. Another key point is that antibiotic resistance genes that mediate the MLS_B-resistance phenotype are found in mobile-genetic elements (MGEs) and, in consequence, may be horizontally transferred to susceptible strains [17]. In Latin America, the resistance rates to MLS_B antibiotics have been reported to be 74% and 81% to ERY and CLI, respectively, among HA-MRSA isolates [10].

In Chile, *S. aureus* is one of the main etiological agents in health care-associated infections (HAIs) [18]. Specifically, it is the main cause of surgical wound infections (27%), and the second cause of pneumonia associated to invasive mechanical ventilation (21%). Likewise, it is involved in bloodstream infections (18%) and infections of the central nervous system (18%) [18]. Despite these data, the MLS_B-resistance phenotype among HA- and CA-MRSA is still unknown among Chilean isolates. Therefore, the aim of our study was to detect and characterize the MLS_B- and MS_B-resistance phenotypes among HA-MRSA and CA-MRSA isolates collected between 2007 and 2017 from the *S. aureus* surveillance program of the National Institute of Public Health of Chile (ISP).

2. Results

2.1. Molecular Characterization of MRSA Isolates

All HA-MRSA (32) and CA-MRSA (36) isolates were resistant to FOX and *mecA* positive. For HA-MRSA, the Staphylococcal Cassette Chromosome *mec* (SCC*mec*) analysis revealed the presence of the Type I and Type II elements in 27 (84.4%) and 5 (15.6%) isolates, respectively. In addition, in all isolates classified as HA-MRSA, the absence of the *pvl* gene was confirmed. On the other hand, in all CA-MRSA (36), the *pvl* gene and the type IV SSC*mec* cassette were detected. Of these, 24 (66.7%) harbored the cassette subtype SSC*mec* IVc, whereas 11 (30.5%), and 1 (2.8%) amplified for the subtypes IVa and IVb, respectively; therefore, they were confirmed as CA-MRSA.

The MLST analyses of HA-MRSA showed that 27 (84.4%) isolates belonged to ST5 and 5 (15.6%) to ST105, whereas most CA-MRSA isolates belonged to the ST8 (27/36) (Table 1).

Table 1. Sequence types (ST) of methicillin-resistant *Staphylococcus aureus* strains isolated in Chile.

	ST 5	ST 8	ST 30	ST 105	ST 868	ST 923	ST 2802	Total
HA-MRSA	27	0	0	5	0	0	0	32
CA-MRSA	1	28	4	0	1	1	1	36

2.2. *Antimicrobial Susceptibility Testing*

The antibiotic resistance profiles were determined for both HA-MRSA and CA-MRSA isolates (Table 2). All isolates (32) of HA-MRSA were resistant to macrolides and to CLI. Moreover, 2 isolates (2/32) (6.3%) were also resistant to CHL and 1 isolate (1/32) (3.1%) to RIF. In the case of CA-MRSA, 9 isolates (9/36) (25%) were resistant to ERY, AZM and CLR, and one isolate was resistant to ERY and AZT (2.8%), but all were susceptible to CLI, CHL, and RIF (Table 2). All HA-MRSA, and CA-MRSA isolates were susceptible to LZD, VAN, DAP, and SXT (Table 3). Furthermore, the iMLS mechanism was detected in none of the two groups of MRSA isolates.

Table 2. Antibiotic resistance profiles among methicillin-resistant *Staphylococcus aureus* strains isolated in Chile.

Resistance Profiles					HA-MRSA *	CA-MRSA *
CLI	ERY	AZM	CLR	CHL	2 (6.3)	0
CLI	ERY	AZM	CLR		29 (90.6)	0
CLI	ERY	AZM	CLR	RIF	1 (3.1)	0
ERY	AZM	CLR			0	9 (25.0)
ERY	AZM				0	1 (2.8)
		All susceptible			0	26 (72.2)

*** No. of isolates (percentage), CLI**: clindamycin, **ERY**: erythromycin, **AZM**: azithromycin, **CLR**: clarithromycin, **CHL**: chloramphenicol, **RIF**: rifampicin; **HA-MRSA:** Hospital-acquired methicillin-resistant *Staphylococcus aureus;* **CA-MRSA:** Community-acquired methicillin-resistant *Staphylococcus aureus.*

Table 3. Minimum-inhibitory concentration (μg/mL) of some antimicrobials against methicillin-resistant *Staphylococcus aureus* strains isolated in Chile.

Antimicrobials	MIC_{50}	MIC_{90}
Linezolid	2	2
Vancomycin	1	1
Daptomycin	0.25	0.25

The HA-MRSA group showed more extended resistance profiles than CA-MRSA. Among the HA-MRSA, the most prevalent resistance profile was CLI-ERY-AZM-CLR, with 90.6% of isolates. On the other hand, in the CA-MRSA group, the most prevalent antibiotic resistance profile was ERY, AZM, and CLR, with 25% of isolates.

2.3. *Prevalence of msrA and erm Genes*

The *ermA* gene was amplified in 28 (87.5%) HA-MRSA isolates compared with 6 (16.7%) in CA-MRSA ($p < 0.001$). Additionally, the *ermC* gene was found in 2 (6.3%) of HA-MRSA and in none of CA-MRSA isolates ($p > 0.05$), and the *ermB* gene was detected in none of the isolates. On the other hand, *msrA* was detected in 11 (30.6%) of the CA-MRSA isolates, but in none of the HA-MRSA ($p < 0.005$) (Table 4).

Table 4. Antibiotic resistance, and presence of resistance genes in methicillin-resistant *Staphylococcus aureus* strains isolated in Chile.

	Percentage of Resistant Isolates to:						Percentage of Resistance Genes:			
	CLI	**ERY**	**AZM**	**CLR**	**CHL**	**RIF**	*ermA*	*ermB*	*ermC*	*msrA*
HA-MRSA	100	100	100	100	6.3	3.1	87.5	0	0	0
CA-MRSA	0	27.8	27.8	25	0	0	16.7	0	6.3	30.6

CLI: clindamycin, **ERY**: erythromycin, **AZM**: azithromycin, **CLR**: clarithromycin, **CHL**: chloramphenicol, **RIF**: rifampicin; **HA-MRSA:** Hospital-acquired methicillin-resistant *Staphylococcus aureus;* **CA-MRSA:** Community-acquired methicillin-resistant *Staphylococcus aureus.*

3. Discussion

In recent years, we have observed an increased resistance to antibiotics, especially in those used for the treatment of serious infections associated with health care. MLS_B group are antibiotics commonly used to treat skin and soft tissue infections caused by CA-MRSA [11]. The present study reports percentages of resistance to antibiotics in the MLS_B group $\geq$90% in HA-MRSA. This finding agrees with the results of previous studies carried out with strains collected in Chile [10,19]. Besides, 20% of strains of CA-MRSA were resistant to MLS_B group. These results show lower rates of resistance to these antibiotics in comparison to the official reports of the National Institute of Public Health of Chile (20% v/s 29%, respectively). On the other hand, our results showed higher values than previous reports that included strains isolated in Latin America, among both HA-MRSA (81% for ERY and 74% for CLI) and CA-MRSA [9,10,20–24].

Among the isolates included in this work, the predominant phenotype was the cMLS_B phenotype. Molecular characterization of 68 MLSB-resistant MRSA revealed that among HA-MRSA, 87.5% were positive for *ermA*. However, in the CA-MRSA strains, 16.7% were positive for *ermA*, 6.3% for *ermC*, and 30.6% for *msrA*. The main mechanism of resistance to macrolides in CA-MRSA is mediated by the presence of the *msrA* gene, which results agree with previously published data [25].

Our results are in agreement with previous reports about the predominance of SCC*mec* type I-ST5 in HA-MRSA in Chile with classic resistance profiles of the Chilean/Cordobes clone that has a marked presence in hospitals of our country [10,26], and isolates of type IV-ST8 in CA-MRSA in Latin America, related to the USA-300 clone [10,19]. On the other hand, the dichotomy regarding the presence of MLS_B or MS_B resistance among HA-MRSA isolates highlights compared with CA-MRSA (97% vs approximately 25%, reaching statistical significance, $p < 0.005$). However, it is important to emphasize that these findings, which are consistent with the classic concept that hospital isolates of MRSA are multi-resistant and the community-based multi-susceptible and only resistant to β-lactams, should be monitored, since 20% of the isolates of CA-MRSA were resistant to antibiotics in this group, that is, 1 over 5 isolates were not widely susceptible. Accordingly, it is important to perform the proper laboratory detection of these phenotypes to analyze these isolates, since if the criterion of resistance to methicillin and broad susceptibility is the method of choice, other families, including those of the MLS_B group, could obtain biased results.

All the strains analyzed are susceptible to VAN, LZD, DAP, and SXT, keeping these antibiotics as an alternative treatment within the therapeutic arsenal available in Chile, which is consistent with previous reports [10,18].

In summary, despite the higher frequency of the cMLS_B phenotype than iMLS_B in this study, we recommend performing the D test to identify clindamycin-induced resistance and guide therapeutic procedures in both HA-MRSA and CA-MRSA. Likewise, it is not recommended ruling out the submission of suspected CA-MRSA strains in surveillance programs based exclusively on the criterion of resistance only to β-lactams.

4. Materials and Methods

4.1. MRSA Isolates

Thirty-two non-repetitive HA-MRSA isolates recovered from eight Chilean cities between 2007 and 2017 (Table 5), and thirty-six CA-MRSA isolates collected in ten Chilean cities between 2012 and 2017 (Table 6) were included in this study. All isolates were selected from the biorepository maintained by the National Institute of Public Health of Chile (ISP), Santiago, Chile. All isolates were cryo-preserved at −80 °C in glycerol (50% v/v) and trypticase broth (2:1). The ISP criteria were used to define HA-MRSA and CA-MRSA [20].

Table 5. Hospital-acquired methicillin-resistant *Staphylococcus aureus* isolates from different Chilean cities.

City	Number of Isolates
Santiago	15
Rancagua	2
Talca	1
Concepción	2
Los Ángeles	1
Temuco	3
Osorno	1
Puerto Montt	7
Total	**32**

Table 6. Community-acquired methicillin-resistant *Staphylococcus aureus* isolates from various Chilean cities.

City	Number of Isolates
Valparaíso	1
Viña del Mar	1
Santiago	14
Rancagua	2
Talca	1
Concepción	5
Osorno	1
Los Ángeles	1
Temuco	3
Puerto Montt	7
Total	**36**

4.2. Antimicrobial Susceptibility Testing

The cefoxitin test (FOX, 30 µg) for methicillin resistance detection, D-test, $iMLS_B$, $cMLS_B$, and MS phenotypes detection and antibiotics susceptibility determination, were performed by disk diffusion method on Mueller–Hinton agar following the CLSI recommendations and suggested breakpoints (2018) [27–29]. The antibiotics tested were erythromycin (ERY, 15 µg), clarithromycin (CLR, 15 µg), azithromycin (AZM, 15 µg), clindamycin (CLI, 2 µg), chloramphenicol (CHL, 30 µg), rifampicin (RIF, 5 µg), and trimethoprim/sulfamethoxazole (SXT, 25 µg).

The minimal inhibitory concentrations (MICs) of linezolid (LZD), vancomycin (VAN), and daptomycin (DAP) were determined using the broth microdilution method, according to CLSI guidelines and recommended breakpoints [28,29].

4.3. Characterization of MRSA Isolates

The presence of *mecA*, *pvl* in MRSA isolates, and the detection and characterization of the SCC*mec* element were performed by PCR-based protocols, as previously described [30–32]. Sequence types (ST) were obtained according to Opazo-Capurro et al. (2019), using the Pasteur's scheme STs employing the bioinformatic tools available at the Center for Genomic Epidemiology (CGE) server (http://www.genomicepidemiology.org/, accessed on 13 March 2022) [33].

4.4. Molecular Detection of Antibiotic Resistance Genes

The detection of genes involved in the MLS_B (*ermA*, *ermB and ermC*) and MS_B (*msrA*) phenotypes were screened by conventional PCR according to protocols and primers previously described [34] (Supplementary Materials, Table S1).

4.5. Statistical Analyses

Pearson's chi-squared test was used to determine associations between antibiotic resistance profiles, MLS_B resistance genes, and MRSA types (CA or HA-MRSA). This was achieved utilizing the IBM SPSS Statistics version 23.0 software (SPSS Inc, Chicago, IL, USA), establishing statistical significance at $p < 0.05$ [35].

5. Conclusions

In Chile, in isolates of HA-MRSA, there is an evident predominance of ST5-SCC*mec* I, a Chilean/Cordobes clone, characteristically multiresistant, which includes resistance to antibiotics from the MLS_B group; and susceptible to SXT and RIF. On the other hand, at the community level (CA-MRSA), there is an emergency of ST8-SCC*mec* IV, related to clone USA 300. Thus, microbiological surveillance of these isolates at the nosocomial level is required to verify whether the Chilean/Cordobes clone will be replaced by this community clone in Chile, and to monitor whether the latter will continue to increase its resistance to non-beta-lactam antibiotics, such as those of the MLS_B group.

Supplementary Materials: The following supporting information can be downloaded at: https://www.mdpi.com/article/10.3390/antibiotics11081000/s1. Table S1: Primers used in this study.

Author Contributions: Conceptualization: M.Q.-A., A.A.-R., S.M.-M., A.O.-C., H.B.-T., G.G.-R.; methodology; software: M.Q.-A., A.A.-R., C.C., D.M., P.S.; validation: formal analysis: M.Q.-A.; data curation, M.Q.-A., A.A.-R., A.O.-C.; writing—original draft preparation: M.Q.-A.; writing—review and editing: M.Q.-A., A.A.-R., A.O.-C., S.M.-M., H.B.-T., J.M.M., J.C.H., G.G.-R.; visualization: M.Q.-A., A.O.-C., G.G.-R.; supervision: G.G.-R.; project administration: A.A.-R., G.G.-R. All authors have read and agreed to the published version of the manuscript.

Funding: This research was supported by Universidad de Concepción, Grant VRID N° 218.085.040-1.0IN (A.A.-R.; G.G.-R.; H.B.-T.; S.M.-M.), the National Agency for Research and Development (ANID)/Scholarship Program/DOCTORADO NACIONAL/2017 21171278 (M.Q.-A.) and by FONDECYT 1171805, the National Fund for Scientific and Technological Development (FONDECYT) of Chile (J.M.M.).

Acknowledgments: We want to thank the microbiologists of the Chilean Hospitals and the National Institute of Public Health of Chile (ISP), who kindly provided the isolates for this study.

Conflicts of Interest: The authors declare that there are no conflict of interest.

References

1. Foster, T.J. The Remarkably Multifunctional Fibronectin Binding Proteins of *Staphylococcus aureus*. *Eur. J. Clin. Microbiol. Infect. Dis.* **2016**, *35*, 1923–1931. [CrossRef]
2. Carfora, V.; Giacinti, G.; Sagrafoli, D.; Marri, N.; Giangolini, G.; Alba, P.; Feltrin, F.; Sorbara, L.; Amoruso, R.; Caprioli, A.; et al. Methicillin-Resistant and Methicillin-Susceptible *Staphylococcus aureus* in Dairy Sheep and in-Contact Humans: An Intra-Farm Study. *J. Dairy Sci.* **2016**, *99*, 4251–4258. [CrossRef] [PubMed]
3. Chambers, H.F.; Deleo, F.R. Waves of Resistance: *Staphylococcus aureus* in the Antibiotic Era. *Nat. Rev. Microbiol.* **2009**, *7*, 629–641. [CrossRef] [PubMed]
4. Malachowa, N.; Deleo, F.R. Mobile Genetic Elements of *Staphylococcus aureus*. *Cell. Mol. Life Sci.* **2010**, *67*, 3057–3071. [CrossRef] [PubMed]
5. Mermel, L.A.; Allon, M.; Bouza, E.; Craven, D.E.; Flynn, P.; O'Grady, N.P.; Raad, I.I.; Rijnders, B.J.; Sherertz, R.J.; Warren, D.K. Clinical Practice Guidelines for the Diagnosis and Management of Intravascular Catheter-Related Infection: 2009 Update by the Infectious Diseases Society of America. *Chin. J. Infect. Chemother.* **2010**, *10*, 81–84. [CrossRef]
6. Chang, S.; Sievert, D.M.; Hageman, J.C.; Boulton, M.L.; Tenover, F.C.; Downes, F.P.; Shah, S.; Rudrik, J.T.; Pupp, G.R.; Brown, W.J.; et al. Infection with Vancomycin-Resistant *Staphylococcus aureus* Containing the *vanA* Resistance Gene. *N. Engl. J. Med.* **2003**, *348*, 1342–1347. [CrossRef] [PubMed]
7. Archer, N.K.; Mazaitis, M.J.; William Costerton, J.; Leid, J.G.; Powers, M.E.; Shirtliff, M.E. *Staphylococcus aureus* Biofilms: Properties, Regulation and Roles in Human Disease. *Virulence* **2011**, *2*, 445–459. [CrossRef] [PubMed]
8. Turner, N.A.; Sharma-Kuinkel, B.K.; Maskarinec, S.A.; Eichenberger, E.M.; Shah, P.P.; Carugati, M.; Holland, T.L.; Fowler, V.G. Methicillin-Resistant *Staphylococcus aureus*: An Overview of Basic and Clinical Research. *Nat. Rev. Microbiol.* **2019**, *17*, 203–218. [CrossRef] [PubMed]

9. da Paz Pereira, J.N.; Rabelo, M.A.; da Costa Lima, J.L.; Neto, A.M.B.; de Souza Lopes, A.C.; Maciel, M.A.V. Phenotypic and Molecular Characterization of Resistance to Macrolides, Lincosamides and Type B Streptogramin of Clinical Isolates of *Staphylococcus* spp. of a University Hospital in Recife, Pernambuco, Brazil. *Braz. J. Infect. Dis.* **2016**, *20*, 276–281. [CrossRef] [PubMed]
10. Arias, C.A.; Reyes, J.; Carvajal, L.P.; Rincon, S.; Diaz, L.; Panesso, D.; Ibarra, G.; Rios, R.; Munita, J.M.; Salles, M.J.; et al. A Prospective Cohort Multicenter Study of Molecular Epidemiology and Phylogenomics of *Staphylococcus aureus* Bacteremia in Nine Latin American Countries. *Antimicrob. Agents Chemother.* **2017**, *61*, e00816-17. [CrossRef] [PubMed]
11. Sarrou, S.; Malli, E.; Tsilipounidaki, K.; Florou, Z.; Medvecky, M.; Skoulakis, A.; Hrabak, J.; Papagiannitsis, C.C.; Petinaki, E. MLSB-Resistant *Staphylococcus aureus* in Central Greece: Rate of Resistance and Molecular Characterization. *Microb. Drug Resist.* **2019**, *25*, 543–550. [CrossRef] [PubMed]
12. Steward, C.D.; Raney, P.M.; Morrell, A.K.; Williams, P.P.; McDougal, L.K.; Jevitt, L.; McGowan, J.E.; Tenover, F.C. Testing for Induction of Clindamycin Resistance in Erythromycin-Resistant Isolates of *Staphylococcus aureus*. *J. Clin. Microbiol.* **2005**, *43*, 1716–1721. [CrossRef] [PubMed]
13. Weisblum, B. Erythromycin Resistance by Ribosome Modification. *Antimicrob. Agents Chemother.* **1995**, *39*, 577–585. [CrossRef]
14. Miklasí, M.; Kostoulias, X. Mechanisms of Resistance to Macrolide Antibiotics among *Staphylococcus aureus*. *Antibiotics* **2021**, *10*, 1406. [CrossRef]
15. Reynolds, E.; Ross, J.I.; Cove, J.H. Msr(A) and Related Macrolide/Streptogramin Resistance Determinants: Incomplete Transporters? *Int. J. Antimicrob. Agents* **2003**, *22*, 228–236. [CrossRef]
16. Drinkovic, D.; Fuller, E.R.; Shore, K.P.; Holland, D.J.; Ellis-Pegler, R. Clindamycin Treatment of *Staphylococcus aureus* Expressing Inducible Clindamycin Resistance. *J. Antimicrob. Chemother.* **2001**, *48*, 315–316. [CrossRef] [PubMed]
17. Feßler, A.T.; Wang, Y.; Wu, C.; Schwarz, S. Mobile Macrolide Resistance Genes in Staphylococci. *Plasmid* **2018**, *99*, 2–10. [CrossRef]
18. Otaíza, F.; Orsini, M.; Pohlenz, M.; Tarride, T. Informe de Vigilancia de Infecciones Asociadas a la Atención en Salud. 2017. Available online: https://www.minsal.cl/wpcontent/uploads/2015/09/informe-vigilancia-2017.pdf (accessed on 13 March 2022).
19. Medina, G.; Egea, A.L.; Otth, C.; Otth, L.; Fernandez, H.; Bocco, J.L.; Wilson, M.; Sola, C. Molecular Epidemiology of Hospital-Onset Methicillin-Resistant *Staphylococcus aureus* Infections in Southern Chile. *Eur. J. Clin. Microbiol. Infect. Dis.* **2013**, *32*, 1533–1540. [CrossRef]
20. Instituto de Salud Pública de Chile. *Vigilancia de Staphylococcus aureus Meticilina Resistente Adquirido en la Comunidad*; Instituto de Salud Pública de Chile: Santiago de Chile, Chile, 2017; Volume 7. Available online: https://www.ispch.cl/sites/default/files/BoletinStahylococcusResistente-20062018A%20(1).pdf (accessed on 13 March 2022).
21. Pardo, L.; Machado, V.; Cuello, D.; Aguerrebere, P.; Seija, V.; Braga, V.; Varela, G. Macrolide-Lincosamide-Streptogramin B Resistance Phenotypes and Their Associated Genotypes in *Staphylococcus aureus* Isolates from a Tertiary Level Public Hospital of Uruguay. *Rev. Argent. Microbiol.* **2020**, *52*, 202–210. [CrossRef]
22. Reyes, J.; Hidalgo, M.; Díaz, L.; Rincón, S.; Moreno, J.; Vanegas, N.; Castañeda, E.; Arias, C.A. Characterization of Macrolide Resistance in Gram-Positive Cocci from Colombian Hospitals: A Countrywide Surveillance. *Int. J. Infect. Dis.* **2007**, *11*, 329–336. [CrossRef]
23. Reyes, J.; Rincón, S.; Díaz, L.; Panesso, D.; Contreras, G.A.; Zurita, J.; Carrillo, C.; Rizzi, A.; Guzmán, M.; Adachi, J.; et al. Dissemination of Methicillin-Resistant *Staphylococcus aureus* (MRSA), USA300 Sequence Type 8 Lineage in Latin-America. *Clin. Infect. Dis.* **2009**, *49*, 1861. [CrossRef] [PubMed]
24. Egea, A.L.; Gagetti, P.; Lamberghini, R.; Faccone, D.; Lucero, C.; Vindel, A.; Tosoroni, D.; Garnero, A.; Saka, H.A.; Galas, M.; et al. New Patterns of Methicillin-Resistant *Staphylococcus aureus* (MRSA) Clones, Community-Associated MRSA Genotypes Behave like Healthcare-Associated MRSA Genotypes within Hospitals, Argentina. *Int. J. Med. Microbiol.* **2014**, *304*, 1086–1099. [CrossRef] [PubMed]
25. Planet, P.J.; Diaz, L.; Kolokotronis, S.O.; Narechania, A.; Reyes, J.; Xing, G.; Rincon, S.; Smith, H.; Panesso, D.; Ryan, C.; et al. Parallel Epidemics of Community-Associated Methicillin-Resistant *Staphylococcus aureus* USA300 Infection in North and South America. *J. Infect. Dis.* **2015**, *212*, 1874–1882. [CrossRef] [PubMed]
26. Vega, F.; Alarcón, P.; Domínguez, M.; Bello, H.; Riedel, G.; Mella, S.; Aguayo, A.; González-Rocha, G. Aislamiento de *Staphylococcus aureus* Hetero-Resistente a Vancomicina En Hospital Clínico Regional de Concepción, Chile. *Revista chilena de infectología* **2015**, *32*, 588–590. [CrossRef]
27. Clinical and Laboratory Standards Institute. *Performance Standards for Antimicrobial Disk Susceptibility Tests: Approved Standard*; Clinical and Laboratory Standards Institute: Wayne, PA, USA, 2003; Volume 23, ISBN 1562384856.
28. Clinical and Laboratory Standards Institute (CLSI). *Methods for Dilution Antimicrobial Susceptibility Tests for Bacteria That Grow Aerobically; Approved Standard—Ninth Edition*, 11th ed.; CLSI Document M07-A9; CLSI: Wayne, PA, USA, 2018; ISBN 1-56238-836-3.
29. Clinical and Laboratory Standards Institute (CLSI). *Performance Standards for Antimicrobial Susceptibility Testing; Twenty-Fifth Informational Supplement*, 30th ed.; CLSI Document M100; CLSI: Wayne, PA, USA, 2020; ISBN 978-1-68440-066-9.
30. Zhang, K.; McClure, J.A.; Conly, J.M. Enhanced Multiplex PCR Assay for Typing of *Staphylococcal* Cassette Chromosome *mec* Types I to V in Methicillin-Resistant *Staphylococcus aureus*. *Mol. Cell. Probes* **2012**, *26*, 218–221. [CrossRef]
31. Kondo, Y.; Ito, T.; Ma, X.X.; Watanabe, S.; Kreiswirth, B.N.; Etienne, J.; Hiramatsu, K. Combination of Multiplex PCRs for Staphylococcal Cassette Chromosome *mec* Type Assignment: Rapid Identification System for *mec*, *ccr*, and Major Differences in *Junkyard* Regions. *Antimicrob. Agents Chemother.* **2007**, *51*, 264–274. [CrossRef]

32. Lina, G.; Piémont, Y.; Godail-Gamot, F.; Bes, M.; Peter, M.-O.; Gauduchon, V.; Vandenesch, F.; Etienne, J. Involvement of Panton-Valentine Leukocidin-Producing *Staphylococcus aureus* in Primary Skin Infections and Pneumonia. *Clin. Infect. Dis.* **1999**, *29*, 1128–1132. [CrossRef]
33. Opazo-Capurro, A.; Higgins, P.G.; Wille, J.; Seifert, H.; Cigarroa, C.; González-Muñoz, P.; Quezada-Aguiluz, M.; Domínguez-Yévenes, M.; Bello-Toledo, H.; Vergara, L.; et al. Genetic Features of Antarctic *Acinetobacter radioresistens* Strain A154 Harboring Multiple Antibiotic-Resistance Genes. *Front. Cell. Infect. Microbiol.* **2019**, *9*, 328. [CrossRef]
34. Dorneanu, O.S.; Lunca, C.; Nastase, E.V.; Tuchilus, C.G.; Vremera, T.; Iancu, L.S. Detection of Aminoglycoside and Macrolide Resistance Mechanisms in Methicillin-Resistant *Staphylococcus aureus*. *Rev. Med. Chir. Soc. Med. Nat. Iasi* **2016**, *120*, 886–891.
35. Jara, D.; Bello-Toledo, H.; Domínguez, M.; Cigarroa, C.; Fernández, P.; Vergara, L.; Quezada-Aguiluz, M.; Opazo-Capurro, A.; Lima, C.A.; González-Rocha, G. Antibiotic Resistance in Bacterial Isolates from Freshwater Samples in Fildes Peninsula, King George Island, Antarctica. *Sci. Rep.* **2020**, *10*, 3145. [CrossRef]

MDPI AG
Grosspeteranlage 5
4052 Basel
Switzerland
Tel.: +41 61 683 77 34

Antibiotics Editorial Office
E-mail: antibiotics@mdpi.com
www.mdpi.com/journal/antibiotics

www.ingramcontent.com/pod-product-compliance
Lightning Source LLC
Chambersburg PA
CBHW062104220926
51850CB00010B/2884
* 9 7 8 3 7 2 5 8 5 1 5 5 3 *